SO, YOU'RE CRAZY TOO?

AMBER PORTWOOD

Post Hill
PRESS

A POST HILL PRESS BOOK
ISBN: 978-1-63758-147-6
ISBN (eBook): 978-1-63758-148-3

So, You're Crazy Too?
© 2022 by Amber Portwood
All Rights Reserved

Cover illustration by Michael Derry

This is a work of nonfiction. All people, locations, events, and situations are portrayed to the best of the author's memory.

Post Hill Press
New York • Nashville
posthillpress.com

Published in the United States of America
1 2 3 4 5 6 7 8 9 10

To all of the beautiful souls out there: if you're not going to read this book from the first page to the last page, don't buy it. The only true story is the whole story.
Love, Amber

For Leah and James:
Anything is possible! Just like your grandfather said:
"It's never too late to change." – Shawn Portwood Sr
We are not a family that gives up on each other or anyone!

CONTENTS

PROLOGUE: WHO IS AMBER PORTWOOD?

I've always looked at myself
From the inside out.
Is that psychotic?
Ever since I was a little girl,
I have felt this as well.
I believe I've always known who I am.
Proud, brave, obnoxious, loud, fearless,
heartless, loving, and kind.
I don't need to find myself anymore
Because I knew all along.

Who am I?

This is a question I have had a hard time answering for most of my life and have only recently figured out. Which is odd, given the fact that I can watch countless hours of myself living my life on past TV episodes: growing up, being a new mom, fighting, mothering, and loving. It's all out there for the world to see, the best and worst of me. My love of prescription opioids clouded my memory, my judgment, and my self-awareness for years.

But I have been sober for some time now, and I can honestly say it has been a struggle coming to terms with the true core of my existence: To begin with, I am—somewhat severely, and certainly clinically—mentally ill.

My diagnoses are varied, and one does not outweigh or counterbalance the rest. The only mental illness I have suffered that has fully gone away was the postpartum depression that hit me like a sledgehammer six months after the birth of my son. Although this episode likely caused one of my most infamous and life-altering experiences, it passed, and I can cross this off the list of the mental illnesses that affected the better part of my life up until now.

So, who am I?

I am bipolar. I have been diagnosed specifically with bipolar II disorder. For me, before I was properly treated, this means my moods swung drastically. I would have long periods of hypomania and even longer periods of severe depression. I have spent my entire life until recently living between extremes, going from the life of the party to a virtual shut-in. Prescription medication can keep this condition under control, but with my history of drug abuse, finding the right medication was a struggle. Of course, medication can take you only so far in the fight against mental illness. I had to find the right psychiatrist and discover ways to calm myself down, to create new methods of battling the demons that have been inside me since I was a little girl.

So, who am I?

I am someone that suffers from borderline personality disorder. I used to cut myself just to watch my skin bleed. I have attempted suicide on several occasions. Before I got my neuroses under control, I would have constant thoughts of self-harm and uncontrollable anger and sadness. This, along with the periods of mania and depression that come with bipolar, was a dangerous and volatile way to live. My illnesses competed with each other; they would hide each other. Some days they would play in my brain like heavy metal, some days muted like elevator music. But for many years they were always there, affecting my actions, egging me on, holding me back. This is how I lived.

So, who am I?

I am anxious. I have been diagnosed with severe anxiety disorder, and this is something I have dealt with for as long as I can remember. Anxiety can prevent me from leaving my house. It can stop me from sleeping. Anxiety affects my relationships and my ability to cope with normal situations; there is not one area of my life that has not been somehow altered because of my overwhelming sense of anxiety. Again, the only way to live a semi-healthy life with my level of anxiety is with intense psychotherapy, calming methods, and prescribed medication.

So, who am I?

I have PTSD, or post-traumatic stress disorder. Many people suffer traumatic situations in their life. I am not the only one who has had a sister, and a father, and a beloved grandmother, and a pet die. I have seen dead bodies when I was as little as the age of five. I know I am not the only person to encounter death so up close and personal and more than one time in their life; however, because of my distinct psychological makeup, I am affected by these major life events in such a way that it has rendered me unable to cope, suffering the effects of these tragedies for years on end, made motionless by their impact on my brain. This is who I am, but it is not.

So, who am I, really?

I am on drugs. As has been well documented, I have been taking some form of mind-altering substance or another since the age of nine. With all of my overlapping mental illnesses, the desire to medicate my way out of them called to me from an early age, and will be something I will struggle with for my entire life. Lately, under the care of a brilliant and caring psychiatrist, I have found a combination of carefully prescribed drugs that are helping me get through my days without total mental collapse. I will likely be on drugs, the kind that destroy your kidneys and liver in a way that will take years off of your life, forever. This has been a battle that I might never fully win.

Coming to terms with my many mental disorders, which happen to be four of the major five mental disorders people are most commonly diagnosed with, now that my brain is cleared from drug abuse has consumed the better part of the last few years of my life. Clearing away the mental cobwebs, one by one, through a strict regimen of therapy and medication, other self-imposed calming methods, and coping strategies has given me the space to share my story—my *real* story—and start to put together the pieces of the puzzle that is my brain so that I can finally answer the aforementioned question with honesty and clarity:

Who am I?

I am, actually, none of these conditions that weave in and out of my minutes every day. I am not just some angry, sad, desperate, lonely, manic, passionate, loud, sweet, smart, funny, creative, sarcastic girlfriend and mother. I am what is underneath all of these conditions, disorders, addictions, and traits—those qualities that make me an excellent reality star and give such good material for gossip magazines and tabloid television. I am what you are about to read. I am a collection of poems, ruminations, research, philosophies, stories, feelings, and anecdotes informed by my experiences and my reading. I am an unfinished sculpture and a work in progress. I'm figuring this out as I go along and sharing what I have learned. I am strong. I am beautiful. I am crazy. I am me.

PART ONE
How It All Began

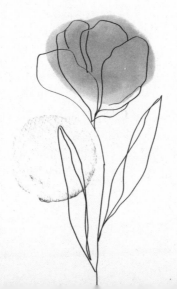

CHAPTER

ONE

Sometimes I look in the mirror
And never really see me.
I see the makeup I use
To cover my face,
The brush to fix my hair
And I look at my clothes
To make me feel
Better about myself.
I always feel better
Covered up fully,
Or playing a part
That's not me.

I DO NOT LIKE MOST PEOPLE. Well, I definitely do not like normal people. I can't imagine saying, "Hey, Sally, let's go grab a drink!" or, "Bobby, how are things down at the Quick Mart?" I don't know how to have mundane conversations. I don't know how to have a humdrum day. I also don't know how to care about anything that is too boring; it just isn't in me to be run-of-the-mill. I can talk about books and philosophy and music for hours. But the minute the conversation gets to how Blake's boss didn't approve his vacation time for his trip to Hilton Head with his family, my eyes glaze over. I don't know if this is a side effect of my mental illness or just that most people have let me down in one way or another my whole life so I have written everybody off as too uninteresting to warrant my time. And it definitely is not because I am a cold-hearted, unfeeling, and uncaring person. I just can't do normal. It just isn't in me.

Lately, I spend the majority of my days (when I am not filming my TV show, *Teen Mom OG*) by myself: reading, writing and listening to music. Sometimes I will hop onto Instagram Live and chat with my fans, whom I actually enjoy and who, for the most part, seem incredibly supportive of a person who has let them down time and time again. But I spend many, many hours each day not talking to anyone. There is a definitely a case to be made that I am too introspective. All of this self-reflection cannot be good for anyone. If you stare at a piece of paper long enough, you start to see craggy edges and microscopic holes and discoloration. That is kind of what happens when you spend your hours watching your life unfold on TV and in the media.

I don't like most people, but I care deeply about the few people I can tolerate. And for some reason, I want to save anyone who needs my help. Even though I can't stand almost everyone, I want to rescue the wounded and helpless. I want to fight for the mentally ill, go to school to learn how to help them, set up places to go for the addicted and suffering, and tell my story hoping that someone might learn from my mistakes. It might not seem in keeping with my reckless and stormy personality, but I really do want to save the world. I had a painful and tumultuous childhood. I somehow survived years of mental illness and drug abuse, and now all I want to do is tell my story as honestly as I can so maybe I can help someone having the same troubles I did. I feel like this might be the only reason I am still, miraculously, on this planet.

I have always known I was different from other people. I prefer my own company to that of anyone else, and I am actually quite shy, something that might be hard to believe for people who watch me on television. I think being on TV since I was seventeen years old has hurt and helped my mental instability in many ways. Obviously, the scrutiny that comes with being on a show that, at one point, had five million viewers is something that would be difficult for even the most normal of people. And I have more problems than most, so my journey has been difficult to watch at times—even for me.

On my show, I am only shown for a few minutes here and there per week, and it is impossible to tell the whole story of anything in that short of time. That part has always been hard for me to deal with: I am honest to a fault, and although I am okay with sharing my life with the world, it is not really the whole truth that is shown—ever. For me, being able to watch my behavior on TV every week has also been a big part of my growth as a person. I find that, for my particular combination of mental disorders, I have always been forced to wear many masks to be able to blend in. I think anyone with mental illness can relate to the masks we wear, whether consciously or not, as part of our coping strategies. I appear on a television network: I wear a metaphorical mask every time I appear on camera. It is a blessing and a curse.

In thinking about my many masks, one might imagine a line of Amber Portwood Barbie dolls. When I was growing up, I was Good Daughter Barbie, Best Friend Barbie, School Barbie, and Cute Little Sister Barbie. Meanwhile, the emotional turmoil that was my reality was hidden from everyone, except maybe my brother. In high school, I became Party Girl Barbie, Girlfriend Barbie, and then, of course, Mommy Barbie. Then came Celebrity Barbie, Domestic Violence Barbie, Jailhouse Barbie, and Knock-a-Bitch-Down Barbie. As my life has unfolded, I became Zen Barbie, Philosopher Barbie, Karate Barbie, Poet Barbie, and finally, hopefully, Doctor Barbie. It is overwhelming to juggle all these personalities, and sometimes I feel like I am not succeeding in fooling anyone, least of all myself.

Over the years I have gotten a lot of comments about my seemingly off-kilter presence on TV. Internet bullies say I slur my words and look like I am going to nod off. "Is Amber Portwood back on drugs?" was one headline I read. No, I am not abusing prescription drugs anymore, but I am on medication that can make you sleepy and slur your words. So, yes, I am still on drugs, just not the kind the haters like to scream about in their headlines to get clicks. To understand what got me to this place, and how to break the destructive cycles of the last decade of my life, my psychiatrist tells me we need to look back at my childhood.

I grew up poor in Anderson, Indiana. I started out a pretty happy kid. My brother and I would put on little performances for our parents in the living room. I sang, and my brother played the drums. I have always had a pretty decent singing voice. I would dance around to songs like "Achy Breaky Heart," and my mom told me when I was not even five years old that I was going to be a star on television. I just had that kind of talent bubbling out of me. She always said I was going to be famous. She was right, of course. I am famous and on television, but this is not the kind of famous she imagined for me when I was belting out songs at a young age.

My mom signed me up for every after-school activity she could think of when I was little just to get me out of our house because my dad was an alcoholic. I was close with my brother and I wanted to do every sport he did, and do it well. I did sports and cheer and I applied myself to everything I tried. It wasn't a stretch to think that I would make something of myself back then because my mom said I excelled at everything I did. She tried hard to get me to dress girly, wear pink bows and frilly dresses, but I dressed like a tomboy. I wanted to look like a skateboarder like my big brother. He was my hero back then, and he still is today.

We couldn't afford a phone until I was in high school. My parents fought a lot. There was tension and fighting that surrounded me for as long as I can remember. When I was very little, I idolized my dad like most little girls. But it didn't take long for me to see that my dad wasn't the happiest of people. He had an explosive temper and yelled at me all the time. He called us horrible names pretty much all day, every day. To this day, if I hear a man use the word "bitch" or the *c* word, it can be a major trigger for me.

My dad drank a lot, and most of his outbursts can be attributed to that. I know this because, in a lot of ways, I have turned into my dad. I abused substances, I have had fits of rage so intense I had no idea they were even happening, and I have done the work to change my situation in life more than once. I know my dad suffered from undiagnosed mental illnesses because my mom told me he was depressed and contemplated suicide. And looking back over his actions, I recognize a lot of the same behavior I exhibit that stems from my mental problems.

Unfortunately, my dad didn't have the money, resources, or education I have today that might have helped him fight his illnesses and addictions.

I grew up very poor mostly because my dad spent all of his money on alcohol. My mom had to work two jobs just to make up for all the money he could not contribute to our household. My mom, my brother, and I would sneak into the house when we got back from somewhere so we wouldn't wake my dad up and have to deal with his temper. I talk to my mom now and she, of course, wishes she got out of that situation much earlier, but back then, there just were not the resources for people to deal with domestic abuse and alcoholism that there are now. My mom was also so consumed with putting food on our table that she really didn't have time for a divorce until, finally, she met someone else who could contribute financially when she physically and emotionally just could not take it anymore.

We were that family, when I was little, that got the box of donations from the church around Christmas time. We were the free lunch family, the family that had to heat our water up on the stove if we wanted a warm bath, and the family that had to miss out on a school trip because we didn't have the ten dollars the trip would cost. But the worst parts of my childhood, without question, were my dad's fits of rage. My brother used to physically fight him. He would wield a baseball bat and swing it around when my dad was in one of his moods. My dad would have my brother up against a wall, choking him during an argument, and this was a usual occurrence in our home. There was a lot of choking going on in my house when I was little: my brother and I would go into his room at night, trying to drown out the fighting of our parents with a loud fan, or (on some of the worst nights) by trying to choke each other out until we passed out. We wanted to sleep and it was by any means necessary.

I know, or I have learned through intensive psychotherapy, that some of my pent-up anger does stem from the hostile environment in which I grew up. I also know there are lots of people who have, or have had, dads who yell or drink. But when it comes to my brain and my specific chemical makeup, I have learned that stressful and upsetting things are harder for me to process than your average person. This complex combination of mental illnesses and addiction makes it even harder to process and grow from bad experiences. It has taken me years of hard work to learn how to put these experiences behind me and react to situations in a healthy and productive manner.

When I was five years old, my little sister Candace died of SIDS. I remember the event more clearly than anything else that has ever happened to me. I recall standing there silently, watching my brother fall on the ground in grief, screaming and crying. I saw my baby sister's purple body covered in blood and on the corner of my parents' bed. I saw the horror on my dad's face that never really went away, especially as he started processing what had happened under his watch, and, mostly because of the lack of information about SIDS at that time, he blamed himself until the end of his days. Other people blamed him because of his drinking. It was the kind of event that can alter a family forever.

My dad had been sleeping in his bed next to my sister. Because he drank a lot, there was a possibility he had rolled over on her in his sleep. They did an autopsy, however, and realized this was not the case. She had simply died of sudden infant death syndrome. There was nothing that could have been done. My mom had to put a headband on her at her funeral to cover up the scar from cutting her head open for the autopsy. I can't imagine being suspected as a cause in your daughter's death. I think this event altered my dad more than anyone. I know we had a lot of strife in our house, but I know so much of what happened was the result of many things: strained finances, an unhappy marriage, alcohol abuse, and my sister's death. It would be difficult for any marriage to survive all of that.

The day my sister died, I stood quietly as my mother rushed in through the door and my sister was wheeled off on a stretcher, leaving behind a bed streaked with dark blood. I didn't cry, I didn't scream, I just stood there and watched. While I was standing there as they wheeled my dead sister on a stretcher out of our house, I kept wishing I could hold her. I wanted to carry her out of the house. And I wanted to just say *shhhhh* so that everyone would be quiet. I wanted to say, *hey everyone, you're not making anything better! Please be quiet!* I was only five, but I knew my sister was not coming back. I just wanted it to be peaceful for our last few minutes together. I wasn't hysterical. I was calm during one of the most horrific events any family can go through. When I saw how everyone else was reacting to her death, this is when I started to realize that I don't process things the same way as most people. And this trait, which can be misconstrued as apathy, has carried through to my adult years.

It might seem on the outside that things don't get to me, but I am deeply affected on the inside by almost everything. I wish I wasn't. I want to be that laid-back, cool chick that lets everything roll off her back. I want to be that tough girl who is so happy she doesn't care what the world thinks of her. And I know it seems sometimes like I don't care about anyone or anything. But the truth is, I care too much about everything. I just have a unique way of showing how much I care.

I remember being on the playground at daycare as a child as young as three, just watching everything around me and not feeling at all like a part of anything. These feelings of isolation have been with me my whole life, but now, as an adult, I have learned to embrace my need to be alone and to feed my curiosity with as much information as I can get on a given day. Not all people who are different are mentally ill, but being mentally ill does make you different. I have been different, in good ways and in bad ways, from most of the people I have ever met for my entire life.

Seeing the dead body of my sister, my psychiatrist now says, has left me with long-term PTSD. The images associated with my sister's death seep into my days and nights as visions and haunting memories. I know that witnessing the aftermath of her death had a tremendous impact on my mental health, and it has taken me years to start to unpack the damage that incident had on my brain. There is so much that happened to me growing up that is taking years to process and compartmentalize, and I feel like that journey of self-discovery is just beginning. Finding out who I really am and why I do the things I do is part of healing, and as hard as it is to revisit some of the more horrific things I have experienced and done, it's part of my growth as a person.

I wish I could say my sister is the only dead body I have ever seen outside of a funeral, but it is not. Death—my own and the death of others—has been eerily present around me my whole life. Once, I was in the car with my mom on her way to work. It was dark and raining, and we saw a car roll down into a ditch. A man appeared and stuck out his arm for help and immediately got hit by an oncoming car. Just after that, he was hit again by a van and decapitated. My mom and I watched the whole thing in horror. It took a minute for help to arrive and we just stared at brain matter in shock. When the police arrived, they told us to turn off our lights and back out slowly, but it was too late: we had seen it all.

I found out later that the guy had been out delivering newspapers. He was trying to put his daughter through college. He was just a good man out doing a good thing. That really crushed me. I think about him a lot even now, and I relive that night in detail over and over in my head. It's not a memory that appears like a movie, like many of my memories. Memories of that night appear like a series of gruesome pictures: a slide show of rolling heads and spilling guts. It is as if my brain is protecting me from having to revisit that horrific night by just showing me glances of what happened instead of the whole terrifying night. I have been down that same exact street many times since that night and I can still see the faint drops of red blood in the road. Just like my mental illnesses, it will likely always be there, a permanent, scarred remnant of horrors.

In addition to the dead bodies that seem to litter my brain, my own death has hung over me from a young age. Thoughts of suicide used to be a part of my daily routine. I first tried to kill myself when I was eleven years old. I often wonder if, when I was attempting to take my own life that young, I was trying to go to heaven to be with my sister. The truth is, I don't know why I did it; I was probably too young to know. But I remember I used a long, windy telephone cord from a telephone that sat in our kitchen unused because we could not afford a phone bill back in those days. I wrapped one end of it around an old ceiling fan in our bathroom and the other end around my throat.

I woke up on the floor. I don't know how much time had passed, but I was in terrible pain. My side and my neck were hurting very badly. A bolt on the ceiling fan had snapped, and all

I could hear was a strange bumping sound as the fan rotated, over and over as I lay on the floor. That fan made that same strange sound for as long as I lived in that house, a constant reminder of my mental state.

It wasn't like I had planned to kill myself for months; it wasn't a cry for help, and I wasn't looking for attention. It wasn't even a carefully crafted plan, as that old ceiling fan was not going to hold up my sturdy little body. I just felt like I didn't want to live anymore. As I look back now, it is clear I was already suffering from mental illness. At the time it just felt like heaviness and, as such a small child without the wisdom of age and desperately looking for a solution to the problem, hanging myself seemed like the only way out. I just wanted the pain to end.

I didn't tell my brother or my parents for a long time. One day I just asked my mom, "Do you remember that creaking sound from the ceiling fan in our bathroom that appeared out of nowhere? I tried to hang myself on it when I was eleven." She didn't seem that surprised, having seen my mental state deteriorate over the years since then. I kept my suicide attempt a secret because I didn't want to worry my family or add more stress and anxiety into their lives. Looking back, I wish I had shared this because maybe someone could have gotten me the help I needed. Since I didn't fix the problems that were underlying such a bold move at a very young age, it became just the beginning of years and years of suicide attempts: not only trying to hang myself again, but also abusing drugs and putting myself in dangerous situations that very easily could have resulted in my own death.

CHAPTER

TWO

In life, I live unfulfilled at times.
Until that new leaf turns over.
I ask for the answers and still, none.
I look for pure love, and still, none.
I looked within myself and to my children
Because that's what was real.
Complete pureness.

ATTEMPTING SUICIDE AT THE AGE of eleven was only the beginning of my lifelong battle with mental instability. I didn't know something was clinically wrong with me at such a young age, but I was self-aware enough to know that my reactions to situations in which I was hurt or embarrassed seemed disproportionate and extreme. I knew I looked at things differently from other people, mostly because I didn't have very many people who understood me. Although I had an amazing mom and a brother whom I was very close to, there was never really a time in my adolescence that I felt safe or protected by anyone. I always felt judged and alienated, and there were very few people who I thought really got my sense of humor and my complicated outlook on life.

When I was really little, maybe six or seven years old, I asked my dad to stop drinking. I approached him and I asked him to stop drinking kind of like I would ask a friend if I could borrow her rainbow loom. He was surprised, of course, that someone so young even knew what drinking was, and I know it affected him that I was aware how his drinking was ruining our family. When he just stared at me, shaking his head slowly, I started to beg him. There were tears in my eyes. He couldn't stop drinking and I think even at that young age, I knew it.

I started to feel severe social anxiety when I was about nine years old. Our house was behind the elementary school, and my parents often argued with the door open and only the screen door shut. Their fights were legendary among my peers, who could hear them screaming and swearing as I got off the bus. Of course, kids can be mean, and making fun of me because I lived in what seemed to them like a war zone became a daily ritual. I was embarrassed of my fighting parents, and I felt like nobody wanted to be friends with the girl who had the parents we could hear yelling from the bus.

My two girl cousins were my best friends growing up, and I was so grateful I had them. We used to compete with each other to see who loved who more, and the younger one, who was closer to my age, was my best friend for years until her older sister became my best friend when we realized we had much more in common than me and the younger one. When things got really bad at my house, I would go and stay with my cousins and my aunt and uncle, sometimes for a month or two until my parents took a breath between fights. It was important for me to have this sanctuary where things were quiet and where I had friends that didn't judge me for my home life. I am eternally thankful for those cousins and that family.

There were some happy memories when I was growing up. When we would take vacations to go see my dad's family in Florida, things almost felt calm. My dad would be on his best behavior around his mom, and my mom, my brother, and I could breathe during a week of blissful normalcy. One time, my dad accidentally set our couch on fire. We threw the couch, still burning, in our driveway and all piled into our car and headed down to Florida like renegades. My brother and I set up a little clubhouse for ourselves in the backseat: we had CD players and would play music like Rob Zombie and sing at the top of our lungs. We had a tiny little black and white TV, and we would pick up the local news station from every town we passed through and inform our parents what was going on in each region like newscasters.

On our trips to Florida, my grandma would show me pictures of my great grandmother, who looked like an Indian princess with long brown hair, perched atop a horse. She told me stories about our ancestors and that we are directly related to the gangster John Dillinger. He was my grandpa's sister's son. That just made my brother and me wild with glee to be related to such a real-life badass. The days I spent in Florida made me forget, for a tiny period of time, the violent arguments in our home in Indiana.

My brother was the closest person to me in the world, and he still is. We would play loud records in his room at night to drown out the fighting of our parents. We bonded over our love of music, and when he would introduce me to certain bands, I would listen to their music over and over again when my anxiety hit just to calm myself down. My brother was a skateboarder, and he embraced everything that went with that, from the skater friends to the clothing. I would copy his style even though I wasn't a good skateboarder and didn't hang out with his group of friends. I felt comfortable with my cousins and my brother, but I was completely anxious when I was with anyone else for most of my adolescence.

One of the reasons I was so anxious had to do with how I was treated by my teachers and peers. When I was in middle school, my teacher gave us a class assignment that involved doing an interview with her on camera. The point was to make us feel comfortable talking about ourselves. It is funny, looking back at this incident, to realize that I would go on to be in front of a camera for almost half of my life. My mom bought me a special outfit to wear for the occasion. This was kind of a big deal. Since my mom worked so much, she typically didn't have the time to get involved with my school projects to such a degree, but on the day before my assignment was due, there was a beautiful, brand-new pink outfit from Old Navy lying on my bed. She had gotten me the whole setup too: pink capri pants with a matching shirt and really cute matching flip-flops. I left my hair down that day instead of the ponytail I usually wore. I couldn't wait to go to school.

In class, the teacher interviewed each of us while the rest of the class waited outside the room. It was a ten-minute interview and the questions were surprisingly very personal. She asked me about my siblings, and I told her on camera about my sister dying when I was little. The class came in, and she screened the interview for everyone on a big projector screen. She wanted us to watch our own interviews and to gauge what the reaction was from the class. She turned off the lights and rolled the film.

As soon as I saw myself on camera, I gasped in horror. Unbeknownst to me, my little brand-new pink shirt had ridden up my stomach and was resting midway up my boob. I was horrified. The class was snickering. I put my head down on my desk and pretended to fall asleep. Hearing the low laughter throughout the classroom, the teacher finally picked up on what was happening and fast-forwarded the video to the end. I stayed with my head on my desk the entire time. The teacher did barely anything to contain the mockery in the classroom that day. She didn't even tell me during our interview that something had happened to my shirt. It was the first time in my life that I realized authority figures, just because they were older than us and were in charge, might not have our best interests in mind.

Another event that occurred when I was younger that made me feel like I was harshly treated by adults and peers was when I was ten years old and my mom bought me some liquid eyeliner and eye shadow from the drug store. It was a big moment for me, not only because we didn't have the kind of money for gifts, but also because I had never worn makeup before. I carefully applied the makeup in my mirror and put little glitter clips in my hair. I looked terrific. I could not wait to get to school to show everyone how cute I was.

When I got to school, everyone made fun of me. They called me fat and ugly. When I got home after school, I took off the makeup and hair clips and got into bed under my covers and stayed there until the sun went down. I cried the whole afternoon. I didn't understand. I know I looked good: my eye shadow was gorgeously sparkly and my hair was combed perfectly. Why was everyone laughing at me? I have never really felt the public's perception of me was in line with my own feelings about myself. I either hate myself and people have sympathy for me and try and pump me up, or I think I am doing great and the world hates me. As I grew older, I found myself desperately searching for a way to feel good about myself and put to rest the echoes of the screaming laughter of my peers.

Self-medicating is very common in the world of the mentally ill. When I was nine years old, I tried my first opioid and it was the best feeling in the world. I felt like I was flying. All of the dark thoughts that muddled my brain were suddenly quiet. My first taste of drugs was a quarter of an OxyContin. After that, I did drugs on a pretty regular basis all through my adolescence. Suddenly, I had all kinds of new friends after being lonely at school for years. I wasn't shy or anxious when I was on drugs. I was popular and the life of the party.

Through middle school into high school, my friends and I raided our parents' medicine cabinets and would pop pills a few times a week to make our days at school more exciting. We had food fights in the cafeteria, skipped school as much as we could, and generally treated middle school into high school like a fun party instead of something serious. My mom worked all the time, and I would have friends over when she wasn't home on a regular basis. I remember one friend scratching our wall with her studded belt, and my mom asking me where an entire pizza went that was in the refrigerator had gone, and thinking it was a miracle I wasn't grounded for my entire teenage years. The truth is I don't know how I got away with the stuff I did when I was a teenager. I was just a resourceful kid with nothing to lose.

My brother left our house for good when he was a teenager, and it was a crushing blow to me. Up until then, he was the only solid presence in my life besides my mom, who was so busy working—and, eventually, hanging out with her boyfriend—that she just couldn't be there for me as much as I am sure she wanted to be. I understood why he wanted to leave: children of alcoholics famously grow up before their time, and he was mature enough to be on his own. Our house was a nightmare on the best of days, but I felt a huge hole in my life the day he packed his stuff and left. He had gone to stay with a friend of his, and the friend's mom was a drug addict just like me. She would send him to the psychiatrist just to get meds for her. My brother had never missed school before and always did well in his classes, but when he stayed with this family, he skipped school a bit, just like me, but nothing like me; I went to about a month of school my entire freshman year. It's hard to top that.

My brother signed up for the military right out of high school, at one of those recruitment things they do in the school gym. He enlisted in the Army and was sent on a tour in Iraq right away. After that, he did a tour in Afghanistan. I was always proud of his bravery, scared for his safety, and above all, filled with love and admiration for him as a person. To this day, when I mess up or slide backwards in some way in my life, my brother is the first person I am worried about letting down. He is my moral compass, and maybe the only person in the world who can talk sense into me. I am not really afraid of anything in this world, but the thought of losing either my mom or my brother is something that keeps me awake at night.

My parents were never home, so when I was young, I fielded calls from the school regarding my absences with ease, and I rarely got in trouble with anyone. I kind of felt like being left alone as much as I was meant my parents didn't care what I did. I was often bored and lonely, and I suffered from crippling anxiety. Doing drugs helped me feel better in my own skin. I felt like everyone loved me when I was on drugs. I was hilarious. I was no longer that weird girl who stayed in her room for hours every day or hid from the mean kids at school (not because I was afraid of them, but more because I was afraid of what I would do to them if they pushed the wrong buttons).

I had no idea at the time that this seemingly harmless distraction of swallowing a few pills here and there to make myself more confident would eventually turn into a full-blown addiction to opioids. Years later, it was Dr. Drew Pinsky who, walking down the street with me in NYC during our first season reunion, told me he was concerned I was becoming addicted to prescription pills. I was shocked. I always thought I had a good handle on what I considered a recreational habit at best. But, of course, he was exactly right: even a clever, smart girl like me was no match for the addictive nature of the pills I was taking.

The most dangerous thing about pills for me is that when I took an opioid, I felt like people suddenly liked me. Who would not want to feel liked? And honestly, that was the first reason I started using so regularly. It wasn't that I was looking for ways to be high or feel good; I actually avoided most other drugs for a very long time. I simply was trying to fit in and become that self-assured, happy, well-adjusted kid I had always wanted to be. That is how it all started, but of course the journey of drug use never starts and ends so neatly and happily. The pills I was taking are so addictive, and the more you take the more you need to feel even a fraction of the feeling that first attracted you to them.

After a while, when you take enough opioids, your body actually needs them to be able to function. That is all you are doing at that point: feeding your addiction so your body doesn't start convulsing and you don't throw up from how much pain you are in when you wake up in the morning. I remember one time I went to stay with my cousins during a really bad time between my parents, and I just took a handful of assorted pills and crushed them up and snorted them, unsure of how long I would be gone from home and scared I would be in withdrawal if I didn't use. It was an awful way to live.

When I was fifteen years old, my dad was diagnosed with cirrhosis of the liver. His drinking had finally caught up with him. At the hospital, the doctor told us he had eight months to live. I was strangely calm about this while my brother and Mom were hysterical. My brother cried so hard he was lying on the floor sobbing. I wasn't that upset. I just had a feeling things would not go that way, and I was right. My Dad gave up drinking and ended up living another ten years. We are a family of fighters, and my dad is no exception. My mom had finally had enough of him, and she had met someone else, so my dad had moved into his own apartment and, for the first time in my life, things around my house were quiet. In retrospect, however, things around my house might have been a little too quiet for an adventure-seeker like myself.

I put myself in a lot of dangerous situations when I was younger, mostly because I really don't get scared of anything. I stayed away from hard drugs like coke and heroin because I prided myself on being too smart to fall down that rabbit hole like so many of my friends. Of course, the rabbit hole I did fall down was just as bad, maybe worse, because pills just sneak up on you. I remember in high school being at a friend's house and some gangbanger tough guy came in with a huge brick of cocaine. He was chopping it up and mixing it with stuff and getting it ready to be sold. These are just the situations you find yourself in when you experiment with drugs at such a young age. All of my girlfriends developed earlier than I did and they were dating older guys who dealt or used drugs. I traveled in that world for most of my high school life, or at least for as long as high school lasted for me.

Despite my dependence on drugs, I held down a job as soon as I was old enough to be employed. Actually, I was working even before I was the legal age to work. When I was old enough, I worked at Wendy's and did very well there. I was about to get promoted to shift manager when TV came calling and changed my life. I was a hard worker and I took pride in the responsibility. My mom drove around in an old Saturn and one of the biggest accomplishments of my life pre-television was that I earned enough money to buy it from her. I experimented with pills but I can say with conviction that I was able to function pretty well for the first few years I was using.

There are so many things that I wish I had gotten help with when I was younger. My mental illnesses, my drug use—all of these could have been curbed at a young age had anyone noticed I was struggling. My mom and my grandma only knew what I allowed them to know, so they could not help me very much. I guess it was my sharp hustling skills that helped me hide so many things I was dealing with from them. In the end, it only made things worse because I was all alone in my suffering. However, having to fix my problems on my own turned out to be something I am sure made me stronger as a person and probably contributed to my ability to finally become the healthy person I am today.

I often skipped school in high school, and my mom, whom I had always had a strong relationship with, started to get angry with me when she finally caught wind of what was going on with me. By then my parents had divorced, something that to me felt like should have happened a lot sooner, and my mom worked multiple jobs to try and support my brother and me. She didn't need the added stress in her life of having to worry about me, and it angered her that I wasn't able to handle so much time babysitting myself.

I always admired my mom. She grew up even poorer than we did. She had to use a blow dryer under her covers to keep warm at night because they could not afford heat. She told me in the winter she would keep a glass of water next to her bed and in the morning, it would be frozen solid because of the harsh Indiana cold. Her family had no working water so they would go out in the rain to shower. They searched for food in dumpsters. My mom would tell me stories from her childhood and they sounded made up, but they weren't. She had a grit and determination under those circumstances that she still has today. I think some of my best qualities, my strength and my honesty, come from my mom.

My mom was a great cook and worked for years in places like the Elks Lodge and various veterans' halls cooking and bartending. She hated being on food stamps and tried her hardest to avoid them most of my childhood. She also had bad scoliosis her whole life, just like me. I knew she was in pain, and I learned a lot about working hard and pushing through pain from her. She went on to get a job in a factory and worked there for the next few decades. She worked nights, and she sometimes worked two jobs, only sleeping a few hours a night. She told me her back pain was so bad she would throw up in her mask at work and have to swallow it and keep working. My mom is the epitome of strength.

When I was fifteen, I had the worst argument of my life with my mom. I thought I knew everything at fifteen. I had been skipping school, taking drugs, and generally letting my mom down at every turn. She tried everything to control me, but she worked day and night and had a boyfriend, so it was impossible for her to keep tabs on me. This all came to a head one night when I was on the phone with my friend. It was 11:00 PM, and my mom asked me to get off the phone. I refused, and we started screaming at each other. My mom, who had never touched me in anger before, pushed me.

My friend's mom heard the commotion on my end of the phone and called the police. The police showed up at our house and my mom, not very politely, asked them to leave. It was mayhem. The police arrested my mom for being belligerent. My mom kicked me out, and I stayed at my friend's house for a few days. The charges against my mom were dropped, but the damage to our relationship was lasting. My dad got involved and asked me to come and stay with him. My mom insisted I leave because she knew she couldn't handle me anymore. Reluctantly, but mostly because I didn't want to face my mom, I went over to his tiny apartment, but I told him I wanted to run away. When he realized I was serious, he called the police and they came to his apartment. It was the beginning of what would end up being a long history of dealing with police officers. I was fifteen years old.

At my dad's apartment that night, the policeman asked me why I wanted to leave so badly. I told him my dad is an alcoholic and that he was dying of cirrhosis of the liver from drinking so much. I said the words with as much anger as I could gather, practically spitting out my frustration with my dad. The policeman stopped me.

He said, "Your dad is dying. He is sober now, and wants to help you. And all you want to do is leave."

When this happened, my dad turned to me. I had never seen him so sincere. His eyes were filled with tears.

"I'm sorry," my dad said. "I am sorry for everything I have done to you. Will you please forgive me?"

And I just broke. I had never seen my dad cry, and I realized what a nightmare I was being to both of my parents. The policeman left and I stayed with my dad, in his living room on a little mattress we found on the sidewalk, for six months after that.

Those six months were the best times I had ever spent with my dad. I discovered we had so much in common. We both loved history and reading. We loved to watch *Scare Tactics* together. We liked science fiction and horror. We would both blurt out funny things we thought of while watching our favorite shows, and it would always make the other one laugh. My dad, despite his depression and drinking, used to take a telescope out to the yard and watch stars and planets with my brother and me. This time spent with him while he was sober reminded me of how much I used to worship him when I was little.

It was always hard to remember those good moments with my dad because there were so many other times when he was drunk and yelling and hitting us. During the six months when I stayed with him, however, I realized my dad had really changed. And I knew I was still going down the wrong path, but I hoped someday I would change too. It took me a long, long time, but whenever I am headed in the right direction in life and I know I am doing well, I think of my dad and how it is possible. People can change, addictions can be overcome, bad deeds can be forgiven. My dad was living proof of that.

Unfortunately, at fifteen I was far from becoming the person I know my dad would be proud of. I was hanging out with all the wrong people: gangbangers, ex-cons, drug dealers, and felons. My girlfriends were actually a pretty good group of people, but they were all more mature than I was, and they seemed to gravitate to the older, rough types. All of their boyfriends thought I was funny: I was a chubby little white girl who dressed like a skater and knew all the words to rap songs. I was easy to have around because I would never snitch and I wasn't judgmental or prudish. I might not have been advanced in terms of my dealings with sex, but I sure knew how to throw down and party if the occasion suited.

A particularly bad group of guys in a gang had taken a liking to me, and they used me as a lookout when they would rob the houses of people from whom they had bought drugs. I would hide behind a bush, or casually walk by a fancy house, and let them know when the owner was pulling up, or when their drug contact was home. One time, they made me come inside a house they were going to rob. I guess they wanted to make sure I wouldn't run and call the police, but they had nothing to worry about. One thing I learned growing up in Anderson, Indiana, was that nobody likes a snitch.

That day, the gangbangers busted into this guy's house and put a gun to his head. They wanted to know where he kept his stash. The guy wouldn't tell them at first, but then they hit him in the face with the gun and his cheek swelled up like a golf ball and he told them where his pills were hidden. The whole scene was fascinating to me. It was nothing like the robberies you see in the movies. Nobody was screaming or yelling, there was no splatter of blood or hysterical pleas for mercy. Everyone was speaking quietly and calmly. There was no negotiation necessary. The man knew he was dead if he didn't give up the drugs, and the gangbangers were as focused on the task at hand as businessmen making a million-dollar business deal. And there I was, in my hoodie and skater shoes, watching a man within inches of losing his life.

Back in those days, I am sure from the outside looking in I looked like just another troublemaker. I was a surly teen who argued with her parents, and I hung out with the wrong crowd getting into the wrong things. I was popping pills and skipping school, and I had no regard for rules or authority figures. It all seems pretty standard for a kid growing up in poverty with parents who were never around. Except that I wasn't your average kid. I was always highly intelligent. I liked to sing and listen to music. I loved to make people laugh. I saw things in a different way than most people I knew. I knew I was special, but it would just take me years and years to figure out what my real purpose was in this world.

CHAPTER

THREE

They say never let
Someone else's bitterness
Ruin your day:
Enjoy your life.
Be happy.
And try to stay calm.
But, what if you're the person
Ruining someone else's day?
Are you a horrible person?

IT IS A WILD THING to watch your own life play out on television. It can be therapeutic, but it can also be a total living nightmare. It just depends on the day. When I was on *16 and Pregnant*, I was seventeen years old in high school in Anderson, Indiana. I was dating my brother's friend. This guy was the second biggest kid in our high school. He was huge. And one time he called me up and said he was in my bedroom going through my underwear drawer. I thought this approach was so weird that I actually fell for this gigantic goofball.

I got pregnant unexpectedly, and because my boyfriend and I were in love, we were excited to have a baby and start our lives together. My family still did not have a lot of money. We didn't have a fancy house or even a telephone until I was well into my teenage years. The only TV we could watch was maybe one show filled with static that we could get by hanging a wire hanger out the window. There were many days as a child that my family wasn't sure how food was going to get on our table.

So when my brother applied to be on the MTV show *Underaged and Engaged* and told MTV that he had a pregnant teenage sister and they asked me to send them a video audition for a new show they were developing, I jumped at the chance. Honestly, I needed the money. Never once did I think that this tape I submitted would lead to a twelve-year television career. Not in my craziest of dreams did I think that sassy little video I sent to MTV that featured my cat lying on my thigh would lead to the life I have now. I actually never wanted to be famous, and I still don't want that, but this is how I make a living. It's a tremendously difficult thing to watch your own life unfold, your best and worst moments, and to grow up watched, and inevitably judged, by millions of other people.

There were not a lot of shows on TV like *16 and Pregnant* at the time. In 2009, when the show began, it was not called a reality show. It was a docuseries, and the producers were dedicated to showing, in as realistic a way as possible, the lives of a few teenagers about to give birth. There was very little intervention from MTV at that time; we were just followed around with cameras and encouraged to live our lives as if the cameras were not there. Years later, the show would turn from docuseries to reality TV.

When the show started, it was a true phenomenon. I was famous overnight, especially in the small town of Anderson, Indiana. Nobody on TV had ever come out of Anderson. I was recognized everywhere I went. It was overwhelming. I went from a typical high school kid to a local celebrity in the blink of an eye. I didn't know how to handle this level of notoriety, and, frankly, I still don't quite know how to handle this.

Reality TV is a big industry, and I make good money. I am eternally grateful for the life this show has afforded me, but things have changed in the world of reality TV. It is a different type of genre now, and more drama is needed to gain viewership. I can definitely say being on a show now is a lot harder than it used to be for me. I miss the camaraderie we had with our old crew. The crew of *16 and Pregnant* was a bunch of kind and compassionate people. I remember having huge "family" meals with the crew after filming, and everyone laughing and joking around. Filming the show at that time felt like home.

The first season of the show featured my boyfriend and I moving into our first house and getting ready for the birth of our baby girl. When the producers came to film me for the pilot of the show, I wouldn't let them film inside my family's home because I didn't think it was nice enough for TV. My boyfriend and I got engaged, and I was all smiles and filled with that new-mom joy. But I was young and I struggled with a host of mental illnesses, some of which had not been diagnosed and most of which were not properly medicated, and I had a pretty drastic opioid addiction that was kept at bay by my pregnancy but that started up again six months after I gave birth. These factors along with my ability to end up in heated arguments and over-the-top outbursts made good TV but wreaked havoc with my life outside the show.

After I gave birth to my daughter, being a mom came naturally to me. One time my daughter had a bad diaper rash. This rash was not your average diaper rash. She was allergic to diapers. It was like she was the victim of an alien invasion. Basically, her skin could not touch a diaper, so for two weeks I held her twenty-four hours a day, letting her pee and poop on incontinence blankets from the hospital that I laid in my lap. I had to change that blanket every two hours, so I set an alarm on my phone and woke up to wash the blanket out every two hours all night long. Every two hours on the dot, at 2:00 AM and 4:00 AM and so on, I would wake up, take the blanket, put it under the hot shower and apply detergent to it, and use gloves and a scrubber to get all of the stains and feces out of it until it was fresh and clean. Then I would hang it over my shower curtain rod to dry. I am a good, dedicated, loving, and kind mom when I am lucid and functioning normally. I am proud of this.

My boyfriend and I had big fights on television, a testament to the true reality of the show, and these fights were not some of my proudest moments as a new mom and a person in general. To experience these dramatic events while being watched by impressionable young people was overwhelming and confusing for me. *16 and Pregnant* turned into *Teen Mom*, and what I thought was just going to be a pilot or maybe one season of a TV show started to turn into a career for me.

Along with being a television star in the small town of Anderson, Indiana, I was making real money for the first time in my life. Unfortunately, during these first years on the show, most of the money I made went toward drugs. And although being recognized everywhere I went sounds fun, it was actually very frightening for a girl with crippling anxiety. Also, my sweet, loving fiancé, who had never gotten much attention from girls before, was struggling with the temptation that comes with being on TV—and failing to resist.

When I look back at that time in my life, I can only really remember the agonizing effects of being addicted to opioids. I could not make decisions properly even though I was a new mom and I was working hard filming my TV show. Back then, when I woke up every morning, I had withdrawal symptoms from the pills I took. I had the chills and my body screamed out in pain until I took the first pill of the morning. It's hard not to look back on those days and relive those excruciating mornings when I could not get out of bed without a pill. I had obligations to fulfill; people relied on me, and unless I swallowed a whole bunch of drugs, I could not function. It was a horrible way to live.

Not only were the viewers of *Teen Mom* watching my problems unfold, but the Department of Child Services and the local police were also paying close attention to my antics. After a particularly brutal fight with my ex when I punched and choked him and kicked him down the stairs on camera, the law intervened. Now in no way do I condone physically attacking anyone. But I have never in my life hit anyone who did not hit me first. When someone hits you once, it is always hard to tell when the next blow will land. Also, at this time in my life, I had no tools with which to resist the urge to fight. When I was threatened or attacked or pushed to my limits, I fought and I fought hard.

On TV it might have looked like I unleashed fury on my ex out of nowhere and that I needed to be locked up in jail. The truth is he had hooked up with another girl, and I was so mad I don't even remember attacking him. Maybe jail is where

I belonged. However, although I had a long way to go in terms of healing the wounds I had suffered as a child and gaining the tools necessary to fight my own demons instead of other people, I maintain firmly that, at that point in my life, I lashed out because I had been hurt by the person I was hitting. It was delayed self-defense—not the correct way to behave, but not exactly the story shown on TV either. It never really is.

When my ex and I had broken up for a while because the fighting was so bad, I was hanging out with a heroin addict and I accidentally got pregnant. It was not an ideal situation. Of course I was not equipped to handle another child. But not being able to handle something and having to terminate a life were worlds apart for me. I finally had an abortion, however, and it was devastating to me. Again, I do not know why I made the decisions I did during this time in my life. I was on drugs and I didn't know what I was doing half the time. I had nightmares about abandoning my unborn child. I cried uncontrollably for weeks afterward. I didn't sleep, and I lost a lot of weight.

Just recently, I heard that heroin addict passed away. I have always felt surrounded by death, and this news made me cry even though I had not seen or talked to him in years. I knew he was an addict and not long for this earth, but we conceived a child together, so I always felt a connection with him.

Back then, things between my on-and-off boyfriend started to get worse. After the televised incident during which I kicked my ex down a flight of stairs, I was arrested for the first (but not last) time in my life. The biggest issue the law had with me, and rightly so, was that my one-year-old daughter witnessed the physical altercation. I was charged with felony domestic violence, put behind bars for two days, and ultimately placed on probation. This whole time in my life was a blur to me. I was grappling with mental issues and self-medicating at an alarming rate. I didn't know how to control my anger, and I had no idea how to curb the drug addiction that was taking over my life.

As a condition of my probation, a probation officer could randomly come by my house and drug test me. One day, when I was sleeping, two probation officers banged on my door until I stumbled down my staircase to let them in. While one of them pee tested me, the other ransacked my drawers and finally came up with a bottle of pills. The bottle was filled with forty various prescription pills. I had violated my probation, and this time it was clear I was going to jail.

As is pretty customary in my life, the story of how I was taken down had many layers. That's what happens when you are on a TV show: only snippets of the truth can be shown, and I am not able to talk about a lot of stuff because of legal or custody reasons. But in this case, when the probation officers busted into my house and searched through all my stuff, I felt violated—plain and simple. On the one hand, it is illegal to possess prescription drugs not prescribed to you, and I was clearly a drug addict that needed to be reeled in. Also, many of the pills in that bottle were prescribed to me; it was actually only four pills in that bottle that did not belong there. But I was on probation and I broke the law. The way it went down, however, seemed brutally invasive and borderline unethical on the part of the officers involved.

One of the probation officers who appeared at my door that day had actually always been very kind to me. One time, she even came to my house and taped the lyrics to the Eminem song "Beautiful" to my door. She highlighted some of the more poignant lyrics and wrote both of our names on the paper. It was so sweet and made me feel like she really understood me and cared about my well-being. She had confessed to me that she herself was taking OxyContin for some knee problem and seemed to understand that I had issues that were bigger than just a young, troubled new mom.

That day, however, when she took me in my bathroom to randomly pee test me, the woman she was with was frantically tearing through all of my stuff. It wasn't that hard to find my pill stash. Every drug addict hides pills under a drawer, but this lady looked like she had just won the lottery when she held up the bottle. There was no warrant, no due process; I was on probation so the state could do whatever they wanted to me. Still, to this day, I feel weird about that situation. Honestly, if they had just asked me, I probably would have produced the contraband. At that point, I wanted the roller coaster to stop. Right then I would have taken help any way it was offered to me, and that is the honest truth. But I was still young, on my own, and struggling with so many issues, and the way that morning played out just made me feel even more unstable and alone.

The bottle of pills hidden under my drawer told the court I was not taking my probation seriously. I had also gotten in a bar fight and was accused of battery and public intoxication just a few months prior to when they found the pills in my home. I hadn't attended the anger management classes I was supposed to attend, and I hadn't gotten my GED, which was a requirement of my probation. I was in big trouble. And honestly, I didn't have the wherewithal, the sobriety, the wisdom, or the good sense to see my world crashing in around me. Life was blurry back then, and I felt powerless to change the direction it was headed.

After a long and drawn-out legal process regarding custody of my daughter, I went over to my ex's house and sat on his porch to talk to him about it. I told him I would pay him a certain amount of money each month, and, on paper, we could have joint legal custody of my daughter. He agreed to this, and our legal battle was over. He assured me I would still see her and be a big part of her life. I was in no condition to care for a child full-time, and I knew it, but this was still a heart-wrenching decision. All I wanted was to have a happy life with my daughter and some peace and quiet from the loud life I was living. To appease the court, I agreed to go to rehab for anger management. Looking back, I should have gone to rehab for drugs, or a combination of drug rehab and anger management, but I don't think the court had a handle on exactly what was wrong with me, so anger management was the program they mandated.

MTV decided to film me at rehab, so I was sent to a beautiful rehab center in Malibu, California, to try and work out my issues with aggression. I was still young, and abusing pills, so I can't say that the rehab really worked, but it was a lovely sixty-day break from the world for me. I would spend as much time as I could during rehab on a white wicker bench with a cushion looking out over the Pacific Ocean. To this day, I remember that spot as being filled with peace and tranquility. I remember exactly how the worn cushions felt when I sat one them, I remember the sound of the waves crashing on the rocks below me, and I remember my brain being as quiet as it has ever been. That's what happens when your thoughts are so busy and loud: when you finally have a moment like the ones I had on that wicker bench, you never forget it.

I made friends in rehab, and I bonded with some of the staff members despite my usual aversion to authority. One of our counselors was a former punk band member, and we got really close. Suddenly, I saw him packing up his stuff. He asked the others to get me away from there because I was getting so upset.

I lost it. I threw the phone I was not supposed to have against a tree and broke it. I cried because I had really connected with him and I didn't want him to go. My phone lay in pieces on the ground, a physical reminder of the fact that perhaps the anti-aggression training (which I was in rehab for in the first place) was not going so well.

One day, a former supermodel and reality star came to give us a talk at the rehab center. She was clearly on some mind-altering substance as she slurred her words and tried to give us advice. I had become close with Dr. Drew Pinsky from my time on MTV, and he had told me I should introduce myself to the guest speaker because he felt we had a lot in common. So, before her talk, I went up to her and said hi, and when I was walking away, I saw her roll her eyes. I was no longer impressed by her presence.

Everyone dressed up for her talk but me. I wore pajamas and slippers with cat faces on them. After her talk, she opened the discussion up for questions, and when I spoke, she pointed out to everyone that the "sun doesn't rise and fall just for you." I walked away. I had had enough of this clearly high older lady trying to talk about drug use. I was in here for anger management, not drug abuse, so I wanted her to leave me alone.

On my way up the stairs, I heard the former supermodel call out to me.

"Hey, Kitty," she said, referring to my slippers. She came running up to me, nice as can be. "Let's exchange numbers!"

I laughed, imagining future sleepovers and braiding each other's hair. I gave her my number, and we actually communicated a bit after I got out of there. I might be a hardened criminal, but I am always open to anyone who shows interest in being my friend. I knew what this woman was all about, however, and I didn't forget her exaggerated eye roll, so I had my guard up, as I usually do.

Rehab ended and I went to live with my grandma. I was still using, so while I was crushed that I wasn't going home to a life with my daughter, I also knew I probably wasn't the best influence on her right then. I was spiraling out of control and I needed help badly. Who knew that the help I needed to pick myself up from my problems would not be from a cushy rehab center with a private chef in Malibu at all, but from the cold confines of a prison cell?

CHAPTER

FOUR

See in Numerology,
Or in the Bible,
3 is to complete an idea, or, let's say,
A time in your life.
There's more to 3, however.
Completion is definite.
0 is eternity and also God.
To me, eternity is the Universe and
The Universe is our God.
0 is to purify.
I'd say, a new beginning.

IN NUMEROLOGY, I AM A master number eleven. This is the most intuitive of all numbers. Master number elevens have an intense level of insight. But sometimes master number elevens lack rational thought. They are impractical dreamers. I am shy but outgoing, violent but peaceful. I am anxious but brave. I am not necessarily religious, but I am highly spiritual, like a true master number eleven. I know I am a paradox. I don't spend money on clothing, but I love diamonds. I can be loving and kind, ferocious and mean. I am aware of my strengths and weaknesses, and I am constantly searching for enlightenment through self-education. And to top it off, astrologically speaking, I am a Taurus. Taurus people are stubborn, strong, intelligent, and uncompromising. A master number eleven and a Taurus. You just don't want to mess with me, I promise you.

I had a fan tell me recently that my belief in numerology was "New Age." That's funny. Numerology was actually begun by Pythagoras, who lived in 569 B.C. So I would say to that fan if I could that numerology is actually an ancient system, and it is not only fascinating, but also shockingly accurate. For me, this way of looking at things was so interesting. For some reason, numerology has always made sense to me, and if that makes me seem like a hippy-dippy New-Age type person, then so be it. I go with what makes sense, and what can help me understand my actions best, and the described ferocity of a master number eleven fits perfectly with my perception of myself.

I can't think of another moment in my life that defined me more than facing a judge and telling the court I would rather go to prison than go to drug court. I wasn't sent to prison; I chose to go to prison. I had a young daughter. If I went to jail, she wouldn't see me for what could be years. And regardless of what people think, I loved her fiercely. This was the hardest decision of my life. But decisions and fighting through adversity? Those are my strong suits. They gave me a choice, and I chose prison. You have to be a special kind of badass to opt to go to jail for what could be five years of your life. You have to be some kind of superhero, you have to have been messed with pretty severely, and you must have had a serious drug problem that you are desperate to overcome if you choose a prison cell over the comfort of your home.

At the time that I was arrested, I was abusing opioids to an alarming degree. I just could not find happiness from anything other than handfuls of little round pills. And even then, it was not happiness that I found, really. It was just relief from the pain I felt inside my head and in my body. The pills clouded my judgment and heightened sides of my personality that were already dangerous and volatile. I was spiraling out of control. When I was ultimately charged with possession of the pills found in my drawer, I was sent to county jail for three and a half months to await my formal sentencing.

County jail is some special kind of hell. County jail is where they send you before they send you to real prison. There are no windows in your cell, you don't get to spend time outside, and there are no organized tasks or activities in which you can engage. You just sit in your cell waiting to hear your fate from the court. Once in a while, they let you out to wash your clothes in the sink or grab an inedible meal. That's it.

When I first entered county jail, I was a heavy drug addict, popping every pill I could get my hands on, and the withdrawal in jail from all of those pills was brutal. I passed out and they had to try and revive me with special smelling salts twice. I saw black spots everywhere and I was shivering and nauseous. They had to call a nurse to come in and examine me. I was in really horrible pain. I felt like I was going to die. For someone who is basically a recluse, I've never had a hard time making friends. I got so lucky to meet nice people who helped take care of me in there. I think that without them, I might have just fallen over and died from pain.

Finally, I was thrown in the drunk tank to get over withdrawal, and I threw up in there constantly. I will never forget the stench of that room, a particular combination of puke and feces. Two nice girls who were locked up as well took care of me while I spent at least two weeks in withdrawal. After three and a half months in county jail, I was brought before the court and, because of my obvious substance abuse issues, I was mercifully not sent to jail; I was remanded to drug court. Drug court is a program in Indiana—well it was. It no longer exists, but when I was in jail it did, and at first it seemed like a gift: a way to avoid prison and also get help with my addiction.

When I got out of county jail, I discovered fentanyl. Fentanyl does not show up on urine tests. A girl I met inside taught me all about that. I had patches of fentanyl inside my cheek when I reported to my mandated drug classes. I was out of control. What had begun way back when I was younger as a way to quiet the voices that had been in my head had become a serious drug habit, and it didn't seem like anything could stop me from obtaining and abusing an alarming amount of prescription drugs.

At one point, I had an idea as to how I could maybe cure my drug addiction on my own. I decided I wanted to join the military like my brother. Before drug court officially began, my mom took me to the place where they did intake for the military, asked for the forms to fill out to enlist in the Marines, and the woman at the front desk laughed at us. I don't know if she recognized me from TV, or just took one look at all the legal troubles we listed on the application, but she said the military could not accept me and seemed confused as to why I would even want to enlist. So it was off to drug court for me.

The courts think drug court is a way to help addicts that have committed crimes but need help with their addiction more than they need to sit in jail. Drug court allows you to stay home from prison and, instead, attend programs designed to help your addiction. I can appreciate the sentiment, but drug court was not going to help a master number eleven who can find a way to outwit any half-baked institution. And that program would have needed a lot of work before it could actually help anyone. In my opinion, the way it was set up was an invitation for an addict to go right on using. I had tried NA, I had been to rehab, albeit for anger management. But still, I was locked up, attending their group sessions and classes, and none of it worked. I did more drugs in rehab than on the outside.

One of the biggest issues I had with drug court is kind of the issue I have with the judicial system as a whole. There is no room for any individual with special circumstances. For me, this meant there would be no alteration of the process for someone having severe mental health issues, and certainly no adjustments were given to me in drug court for being a celebrity. That sounds spoiled, I know. "Treat me differently because I am on TV!" But hear me out. At the time I was sent to drug court, my show on MTV had five million viewers. I had been on magazine covers (the full cover or, more often, in the bubble on the front of a magazine next to an A-list star).

In my small community in Indiana, I was well known. I was recognized most places that I went. This sounds glamorous and fun, but it really was not. I have never seen being on TV as something grand and magnificent. People always say to me, "That's what you signed up for."

Well, it really wasn't. I was young and poor and pregnant. When they reached out to me, I simply needed the money they were offering me. Never in a million years did I imagine this would turn into a twelve-year career, or that I would receive the type of notoriety I eventually gained. I am on TV, I get paid to air my life, and it has always been hard for me, but my job made drug court almost impossible to complete.

I had to report to drug court to attend mandated classes at a painful 6:00 AM—something that was made even more difficult for me by the host of psychotropic drugs I was both prescribed and not prescribed, but felt like I had to take to be able to get out of bed in the morning. To begin your day at drug court, you had to sign in on a form that was public and included your phone number. Right there, I had a problem. Now a bunch of drug addicts had my phone number, and in Indiana at the time, I was a public figure. Not that there is anything wrong with being an addict—I was one myself—but addicts generally aren't known for self-control and discretion.

Almost immediately, I began getting strange calls and texts from other people in the program—mostly men, of course. One guy sent me a picture of his penis. I got asked out on dates. None of the attention was necessarily flattering, mostly because of the unsolicited nature and the creepy demeanor of the calls. I complained to the people at drug court and there was nothing they could do. It was policy. Everyone must put their number on the sign-in sheet. No exceptions.

I am the first to admit I am a big personality. And in the twelve years I have been on television, I have run into people (especially women) who do not like the fact that I am on television. I don't know if it's jealousy or just plain resentment, but I have encountered hatred for no reason other than my job a lot over the years. One woman whose picture on her social media profile showed her and a lovely looking family wrote me and told me she would like to see me experience a very gruesome death. She described my suicide to me in detail. This woman looked in her profile picture like a perfectly lovely mother of two. I don't know why I inspire such hatred sometimes, but I do.

In drug court, there was one woman in particular who worked there who did not like me from the moment we met. I could tell. She just could not stand me, possibly for the fact that I was a well-known person in that area, or maybe she didn't like my attitude. That is highly probable, as I am the first to admit I was filled with attitude at that time in my life.

I did nothing at the beginning to deserve this woman's bitterness, but her disdain became a huge problem for me. She was the person who monitored my pee tests. We would go into the bathroom and I would sit down to pee, and after about thirty seconds she would start saying, "Are you going to pee today?" This question occurred with lots of attitude and many eye rolls and exaggerated sighs. I have been diagnosed with clinical anxiety. The woman pushed every button I had and was literally making it impossible to pee—and in drug court, peeing is mandatory. No exceptions.

Once again, I went to the people who ran drug court. I begged them to put someone else on pee duty. I was not interested in messing up my part in the program. I wanted to pee in the cup. I had too much to lose to fail. But this woman was relentless with me. She had no interest in helping me; she was purposely standing in my way. And the higher-ups could not have cared less. Once again, I felt like the whole program was set up for me to fail.

Two times during drug court, I was sent to jail for not being able to pee. I was given five days in county jail where there are no windows and you sit in a cell lined with grey bricks that look like Legos waiting to be released. If you think I did not badly want to pee to avoid county jail, you would be sorely mistaken.

Unfortunately for me, the woman who supervised my pee tests had it out for me, and because of my severe anxiety, I wasn't able to perform under pressure. I was being set up for failure. But it is just not in my makeup to shy away from adversity or avert my gaze when being stared down. This situation was becoming dangerous for both of us.

Another difficulty for me was that the participants of drug court were required to get a job. I understand the sentiment here. Drug addicts need to be busy, and being gainfully employed can help with sobriety. And, just like having to pee test, getting a job helps show the court you are taking the program seriously and are not out getting into the kind of trouble that landed you in drug court to begin with. However, in my case, getting a job proved to be impossible. I went on interviews. I did as I was told. But who is going to let someone on an MTV show make bagels at their café? Who wanted someone that had received so much negative press working at the car wash? Nobody. I went on interview after interview, and I couldn't get a job. Again, the court did not care. Getting a job was part of the program. There were no exceptions.

Now I admit, at the time, I was probably not making the best decisions or following rules to a T. I was taking a massive amount of drugs—I am talking medical-grade stuff they give to cancer patients—just to get through my days. Going on a whole host of job interviews and pounding the pavement to find a job was likely not on the top of my list of things to do for the day. I did go on some interviews, and immediately I could tell it was going to be very difficult to get a job in my position and with my level of notoriety. I am going to be completely honest here and say I probably did not give this particular task my all; however, I would still like to point out that one of the flaws in the program was that there was no help to be given to anyone struggling to meet the requirements. You would think in a program designed to help drug addicts, allowances would be made and extra help would be given to someone who was on so many drugs the program was proving a challenge to complete. But I was on my own, treading water, thrown before a disapproving judge every so often. I was sinking fast.

Another mandate of the program was that people in drug court had to go to a halfway house. I didn't mind this at all. I felt like the rigid rules in a halfway house would help me get sober. But again, my status as a television personality proved to be a problem regarding my acceptance into any program. Nobody wanted the halfway house that they ran to receive the amount of attention that, at this point, was inevitable if I were to arrive. I applied at a bunch of halfway houses in my area, and every single one of them turned me down. I know this sounds like an excuse. I know I maybe could have tried harder to find a place that would have taken me. If sober, I probably would have banged on every door in Indiana. But back then, these little issues just seemed to add up and make the whole experience of drug court seem impossible to me.

Again, I went to the people who ran drug court to tell them I was having trouble finding a place that would take me. And again, there was no way to bend the rules. No help was given to me at all. At one point, the judge insisted he had told me to call a certain halfway house. When I said I had never been told about this particular halfway house, he rolled the tape. It turned out I was right; he had never given me that instruction. But of course, when we finally called them, that halfway house wanted nothing to do with me either. Still, nobody in the program really cared. I had to go to a halfway house to participate in the program, and it wasn't their problem that no house wanted me. I was being set up to fail.

There was another aspect of drug court that was difficult for me. It just wasn't foolproof enough for a highly functioning drug addict. Pee tests can only detect certain kinds of drugs. I arrived at drug court with fentanyl patches in my cheek and nobody checked. Fentanyl does not show up on a pee test. Many times, I nodded off from the heavy drugs I was on in the NA meetings I was forced to attend. I saw other people nod off as well. Nobody intervened and nobody seemed to care about my individual situation. My grandma attended the meetings with me and agreed that for my personality, they were useless. This is not the kind of help I needed, but the program was the program and I was certainly in no position to make waves.

Another problem that arose for me during drug court was that I had to get my gallbladder out. While this is a somewhat common procedure, the recovery can be painful. And of course, just my luck, I did not recover as quickly as is typical for that kind of operation. Once again, drug court has rules, and they decided recovery from gallbladder surgery should be two weeks. So, two weeks on the nose later, I was expected to attend the classes associated with drug court. This was physically impossible for me to do. I was still in a massive amount of pain from the surgery. Once again, there were no changes made for special circumstances and no allowances made for the severe physical pain I was experiencing. It was their way or the highway. The highway was looking better and better to me by the day.

Everything came to a head for me in the bathroom one day. I was trying to pee. I really was. But my supervisor was taunting me. She was impatient, angry, jealous, hateful, and mocking me at every turn. She made loud grunting noises when I tried to pee.

She rolled her eyes and glared at me. I couldn't take it anymore. I know my impulses are rash. I am aware that once my buttons are pushed, I see red and there is not much I can do to control myself. That was especially true at this point in my life, before I climbed out of the hole I was in and made my life better.

In that moment, I could only pee a tiny amount. I knew it wasn't enough for a pee test. She was annoyed with me, and she was impatient and rude. I had had enough. I was not going to make it in drug court. I was going to go to jail for not being able to pee, and I was probably going to be kicked out of the program for good and sent to prison for five years if I did not fill that cup to the proper amount. I took the cup filled with pee and added some toilet water to it. I slammed it on the sink and said, "There's your pee." I stormed out of the bathroom, got into the car with my grandma, and that was the end of drug court for Amber.

That night, knowing what was in store for me, I tried to kill myself again. I had twenty pills of Suboxone on hand. This is a drug they give you to try and fight opiate addiction, kind of like the methadone they give to heroin addicts. I figured if I swallowed all twenty of the pills, I would never wake up. I took a pill at a time and passed out after I reached about six pills. Throughout the night I would wake up and take another couple of pills. This went on until I finally fell asleep for what I thought was forever. To my dismay, I woke up in the morning. My head was pounding, my vision was blurry, and there were only two pills left in the bottle. I have no idea why eighteen Suboxone pills didn't kill me, but I had court to attend. So I pulled myself out of bed, put on my most fly outfit, and got ready to face the judge.

I appeared before the judge and shocked the court by telling them I was done with drug court. The judge asked me if I knew how much time I was going to have to spend in jail. I told him I was aware it could be five years in prison. There was a collective gasp in the court. I was willing to do whatever time I had to do. I needed to get sober, and drug court was making that even harder than normal for me. Also, I was sure the program was not going to work for me as a whole. I wasn't going to be able to get a job or attend a halfway house, and I couldn't pee on demand. For some people, I am sure drug court worked. I appreciate the thinking behind the concept: people with addiction should not be treated the same as other people in the judicial system any more than the mentally ill should be treated equally. But for me, drug court was a recipe for disaster. I was going to prison.

My ex came with me the day I opted out of drug court. I didn't want my family there because I knew it would be hard for them to see me taken away to prison. My grandpa was not supportive of my decision to leave drug court at all. My grandma, who is a badass like me, understood my reasoning completely. But I thought at the time that it would still break her heart to see me hauled off in handcuffs, so I let my ex take me.

At the sentencing the judge said, "I heard you slammed a cup of diarrhea on the sink." The court gasped. I looked back at the pee test supervisor in the courtroom, knowing she had made that story seem worse than it was. "That's not what happened," I said. The truth didn't seem to matter. I was set up to fail, and I failed. When the ruling came down that I was going to prison, I asked if I could give my ex a hug goodbye. Nope. Hugs weren't allowed. And off I went to jail.

CHAPTER

FIVE

Are we selfish
To think of ourselves
So intelligently?
As if we matter more than another
In a certain way?
What if your burdens or emotions
Do matter more?
We are wrong to think that way, of course.
See, someone always has it worse.
A lesson I am still learning.
The hard way.

AT FIRST, I WAS SENT to a cellblock in the Indiana Correctional
Facility that was for violent felons only. My first bunky was
in prison for hacking up a Mexican man with a machete. I was
fascinated with the complete lack of emotion she showed and the
blackness of her eyes, and I didn't bond with her at all. I don't
like murderers or anyone who harms a child, and I stuck to that

the whole time I was in jail. I would be your friend as long as you were not in jail for either of those crimes.

I didn't really feel fear in prison, but then again, I don't feel fear that much on the outside so this was probably to be expected. As I walked around the prison, I got, "You don't look like you belong here!" pretty often. At this point in my life, at twenty-three, I had been diagnosed with manic depression and a severe anxiety disorder, but I would find out over time that these diagnoses were just the tip of the iceberg. I think many people with mental illness wear a mask to hide their problems, and having been on TV for six years of my life at this point, I was a professional mask-wearer.

The mask I chose for jail was my funny, sweet mask. I felt like this would be the best way to survive what could be years living among these tough, hardened women. Everyone thought I was hysterical. I told funny stories of life on the outside, and I was popular and well liked. There were no fits of rage in prison, no outbursts or month-long bouts of not getting out of bed—not that that was allowed, anyway. If someone came in and cut open my brain, the dark thoughts and constant haunting visions would have had me sent to a psych ward immediately. But somehow, I was able to hide this side of me from everyone during my time in prison.

What seemed like a selfish decision to not be able to see my daughter for what could be five years turned out to be one of the best decisions of my life. Prison was good for me. I got my GED and actually got the highest score in my program. I was a model citizen in prison. I joined the CLIFF Program, which stands for Clean Lifestyle Is Freedom Forever, and they even put me in charge of stuff. I actually taught anger management behind bars. I had friends in prison, and the toughest girls in my cellblock protected me. In prison, people messed with me much less than they did on the outside.

After I graduated from the CLIFF Program, the prison made me a head facilitator, and I was teaching classes for the program while I was in jail. The fact that I was allowed to teach other people made me feel so proud of myself. This was the first time I had been put in charge of anything in my entire life and the first time I could actually see the effects of my help on people.

I met women who were such bad addicts they had ruined everything in their lives just for drugs. I could relate to them, and I really felt like my stories were inspiring to the women in there who felt like there was no chance of success or happiness in their lives after all of the things they had done because of their drug habits. I learned from the women as well about the kind of life I did not want to lead when I got out of jail. I knew I was lucky I was even alive after all the pills I had taken over the years. When I went into jail, I thought my show was over. I had no idea what I would do for a living when I got out. I didn't have a lot of money left from the show, and my mom was even worse off. When I first got to prison, I told her I was craving a cheeseburger, and I had no idea she put her last ten dollars into my account so I could buy one from the commissary. I didn't know what life had in store for me when I finally got out, but I met lots of women in jail who had it much worse than me.

I made friends with two girls who were girlfriends. One was butch and the other was stunningly beautiful. One day, they asked me to stand watch outside the bathroom while one of them punched the other one in the face. They fought for a few minutes and in the end, they had marks all over them. Blood was everywhere. I took rags and cleaned up the mess and threw the rags in the garbage. Nobody cried or told the guards; this was just how beefs were settled in prison. Once I went to the CLIFF Program, I would run into the pretty one in the hallway all the time and she would tell me she loved me and missed me. These are the bonds you form when you experience prison life together. I heard she threw coffee in some other girl's face because the girl owed her food. These girls lived at a special level of badass that even I could not reach.

Another girl I met there used to show me her boobs when I was feeling down. It always made me laugh, no matter how low I was feeling. I barely knew this girl, but somehow, she would find me when I was upset (usually about missing my daughter) and pull up her shirt, and it worked. I felt better. I would get sad about not being able to see my daughter for sure, but I saw other women who would collapse on the floor after they got off the phone with their children, bawling hysterically. The prison was filled with moms missing their kids. Watching a woman scream into her phone and then fall to the ground in hysteria just because she couldn't take hearing the sound of her child's voice is something that haunts me to this day.

I made the right decision to serve my time instead of ramming my head up against the wall that was drug court, but not seeing my little girl broke my heart. My ex said he was going to bring her to see me, but something always went wrong with the paperwork. I only saw her once the whole time I was away. The day my ex brought her to prison to see me, all the girls made such a big deal about it because they knew what she meant to me. I talked to my ex a lot the whole time I was away, which helped until it didn't. I was still so young, and I was trying to hang onto my dream of having a family that lived all in the same house. This dream, however, was not going to come true, although I didn't know it at the time. I was not destined for a normal life, especially with my issues with drugs and my battle against the constantly changing chemicals in my brain.

Prison life, as it turned out, kind of seemed to help some of my mental illnesses. I suffer from extreme anxiety, which on the outside manifests itself in my shutting myself in my home for days on end. In prison, I was in my own cocoon, sheltered from the constant criticism and pressures I suffered on the outside. I had my headphones on all day, listening to music. We called our headphones bitch blockers. They played music over the loudspeakers all night long, and I stayed awake at night until 4:30 AM to hear my favorite song from a local DJ: Kendrick Lamar's "Bitch, Don't Kill My Vibe." During the day, and against the rules of the prison, all the girls would sing "Start a Riot" by Duckwrth and Shaboozey and "Locked Up" by Akon.

However, prison was not all singing and lovely bonding by a long shot. Once I saw a girl get beat up while she was on the toilet. She was sitting all by herself, taking a crap, and some girl came in and beat her to a pulp, and the girl on the toilet barely blinked an eye. She didn't run to the guards, and the girl who beat her walked away. Sometimes I would try to go to the bathroom when I was in there, and there were girls having sex in every single bathroom stall. I had to wait until they were done to go in. It was a different world in there, and I am proud of myself that I didn't get into any trouble and kept my head down the whole time. Prison was cold and impersonal. Most of the time you were just called by your number, not your name. It was actually a relief after not being able to go to a restaurant without someone calling out my name. For someone who had been on the road to a pill overdose, prison was a lifesaver.

What is crazy about my life, though, is when I was at the VMAs a few years after getting out of prison, I saw Kendrick

Lamar standing just a few feet away from me, singing his song "HUMBLE." Dr. Drew Pinsky's wife took a video of me singing the song at the top of my lungs and dancing, right there at the VMAs like there wasn't a soul watching me. We used to sing that song in prison. It was such an everything-comes-full-circle moment. Going to prison was one of the hardest and smartest decisions of my life.

I don't want to paint too pretty a picture of being locked up and not being able to see my daughter for what turned out to be seventeen months of my life. I remember being really sad that I could not see any stars through the window in my bunk because the yard lights were too bright. I cut myself while I was in jail, which was my way of controlling my surroundings. I inflicted physical pain to take the focus off my mental pain. It wasn't really hard to do that prison; you just take the head off of a razor and put it in your hoodie. The lines I made on my body were a constant reminder that, as funny and friendly as I seemed on the outside, turmoil was still simmering under the surface.

Although I was not taking pills, I was also not fully sober while in jail. We would make something called hooch and put it in shampoo bottles. We had to let air out of the bottles periodically so the bottles would not explode, and we called it burping the baby. Fortunately, I was able to stay away from the hard drugs that are also pretty easy to get in prison, especially for a girl who was on magazine covers and had money in the bank. But drinking hooch every once in a while with my friends made me feel normal for a few minutes, and it helped me bond with the girls. Also, I had not learned yet to just live in my own skin without any mind-altering substance. That would still take me years to figure out. I honestly think being in prison laid the groundwork for the person I am, at long last, starting to become.

I was kicked out of high school and sent to alternative school. Then, of course, I dropped out when I became pregnant. While I was in high school, I don't remember attending classes very much. That part of my life is just a haze of pill abuse. So I wasn't sure how I would do on the GED in prison. Amazingly, I aced it. I was the top scorer in the whole CLIFF Program. I loved studying for the exam. Before I was locked up, I had helped my ex study for his CNA, and I think those study skills benefited me in jail. When I called to tell my ex how well I had done on the GED, he didn't believe me—and I can't really blame him, given my track record.

Participating in the CLIFF Program was the first time in my life I was given the responsibility of teaching, and I was trusted to help someone other than myself. I have to say it was addicting. I loved listening to people's problems and trying to find solutions for them. Lots of drug addicts struggle with mental illness, so I could relate to them pretty well. I am a master number eleven, so I am intuitive and empathic. I think these traits helped me do really well in the prison CLIFF Program. But I was still young. Nobody had yet diagnosed me fully for all of my mental issues, and I had never bought into any kind of sobriety. I wish I could say I got out of jail and my life has been stellar ever since, but that could not be farther from the truth.

Thanks to my involvement in the CLIFF Program, and my good behavior, I was able to get out of prison in seventeen months. While I was in prison, I communicated with my baby girl's father constantly. He took money from me to help pay his bills, and we talked about our future. We had had problems before I went in, but he assured me that when I got out, we would be a family again. This dream of mine, that I would finally have a family and we would all be together, kept me going on my darkest nights. I would lie in my bunk looking out at the bright light of the prison yard and imagine making my daughter breakfast in the morning. All of the days of my ex cheating with thirsty fans and lying to me were over. I had cleaned up my act, done the hard thing, and my reward would be our life after jail.

Unfortunately, things did not turn out the way I had hoped. They never really do. When I was in jail, I found out my baby's daddy had met someone. When I got out of jail, I learned she wasn't just a floozy groupie that he hooked up with like in the old days. She was a serious girlfriend. I figured this out in the car with him on the way home from Disney on Ice with him and my daughter, right after I had gotten out of prison. My ex was on the phone with this girl he had been seeing, and they were arguing. The fact that they were arguing so loudly and passionately was the first sign to me that this was not some girl he was just passing the time with while I was away. They were in a real, long-term relationship. And practically the whole time I was in jail, I had no idea she even existed.

After a while, my ex and his girlfriend got married. The girl and I had some things in common, actually. She had some of my good traits, like being able to put up with my ex and being great with my daughter. However, this meant that my dreams of being a family with him and my daughter were over. I was especially surprised by this because my ex had spent some of my money while in jail, and he had constantly reassured me when I was in there that I would get out and we would all be together. This new information, coupled with the very common anxiety that exists for anyone leaving the confines of prison sent my neuroses out of control.

I wanted revenge against my ex for lying to me the whole time I was in prison. As it happened, my ex's best friend had been the only one to send me pictures of my daughter in jail, and eventually he had started sending pictures of himself, shirtless and working out, so naturally I slept with him the second I got out of jail, killing two birds with one stone. I hadn't had sex in a long time, and I also wanted to get my ex back for all of his lies. I didn't have very many weapons at my disposal those days, but I have always known how to use my body to get what I want. This was a satisfying way to let my ex know how hurt I really was.

Clearly, I was sicker than ever when I got out of prison if that was my way of thinking. In reality, I should have been focused on cleaning up my act. At that time in my life, I thought about suicide every day. I stayed away from pills, for the most part, but alcohol became my drug of choice. I would start drinking in the afternoon and it continued throughout the night. I stayed with my grandma and tried to pick up the pieces of my life left behind by being gone for seventeen months, but I felt out of place, disoriented, and distant from the most important person in my life: my daughter.

I tried to kill myself again around this time. I don't even really remember exactly why, which is, come to find out, a hallmark of mental illness: acting without knowing why you are doing the things you do. I do know that I was tired of living. I was giving up on all of my fights, and I was ready to go. There might have been a specific problem that triggered the attempt on that day, I guess. It might have been because I was sad about missing seventeen months with my daughter or because I got in a fight with my ex. I was always fighting and I was just tired of it. As anyone who has as many mental issues as I do can attest to, suicide as a way to end our pain is always at the forefront of our brain until we can gather the tools necessary to fight this impulse.

Before I was going to kill myself, I called my daughter's father to say goodbye. That might look like a cry for attention or help, and it may seem as if I wanted to be stopped, but I honestly just wanted him to know I loved him and my daughter before I left this earth for wherever we go after life. I was confident that my last suicide attempt had taught me the proper way to hang myself, so even if my ex wanted to save me, he would not have the time to do so.

Well, as it turns out, I am just not very good at hanging myself. The bottle of pills I swallowed before I tried to hang myself didn't help my mental state, and so I ended up rocking back and forth on my heels on the hood of my car in vain, and all that happened to me was some bruising on my neck and a trip to the local psych ward when my ex showed up with the police. They put me in the suicide watch wing of the local psychiatric hospital for a week, and I wanted to get out of there so badly that I broke my own honesty-only policy for a week and assured them I was no threat to myself or others.

The psych ward was not so different from jail, to be honest. It had bland, cement brick walls and inedible food that you had to eat at a long table with other inmates. My room was bare and cold. I also got no real help from any professionals in that hospital that would benefit me when I left the psych ward, so I guess I just didn't really see the point of being there. I spent so much of my early twenties looking for things that would help me get out of the trouble I was in, and nothing had worked so far, not even a team of professionals at Indiana's best mental hospital.

After jail, I was shocked when MTV approached me about filming a new show called *Teen Mom OG,* and my first instinct was to turn them down. My sobriety from pill abuse was still new, and being on a TV show and criticized so much triggered my need to self-medicate. I was surprised they even wanted me on the show, given the negative publicity that always followed me around. Something told me to run in the other direction, but my mom and grandma seemed to think me being on TV was good for me. Something about being held accountable for my actions. I think they were just desperate for me to calm down and start living my life as an adult and not a wild child. My instincts to not do the show, however, were probably dead on, because life after prison was about to go from bad to worse.

After I got out of jail, I was still on a mission to find some peace in my life. I had no idea where to begin. I wasn't out looking for a boyfriend, but a few of them found me. I still thought the answer to all my problems was falling in love. Turns out that was the opposite of what I really needed. Unfortunately, being on TV attracts men that are interested in the attention and money that came with my job. I still had a ways to go until I realized how to figure out which men wanted me for who I was and which men were in it for everything that came with being with me.

PART TWO
History Repeating

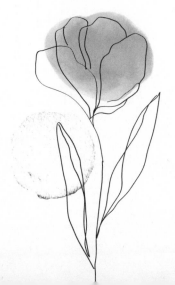

CHAPTER

SIX

Who can you be physically or
Beyond this being we are trapped in?
On both sides,
Good and bad exist
And the energy is still the same.
I can be used to harm or help.
Sometimes, though,
If you choose to have bad intentions
And want some things,
Use that energy to help push
In a positive way.

I HAD BEEN BADLY BURNED BY my last long relationship. My ex had cheated on me, lied to me, and fame turned him into a totally different person than the one I met and fell in love with in high school. So, one might think I would avoid any situations that seemed sketchy, especially ones that involved complete strangers who reached out to me on the internet. But I am really not afraid of anyone, and it is hard to tell me things. I generally have to learn for myself. I am also a deeply empathic person who gravitates toward people who seem broken and can possibly help me reach my life goal: to have a family that lives under one roof, to feel safe and at home somewhere in the world.

I dated a few people right around the time I went to prison. Two of these relationships had ended in pregnancies: an abortion and a miscarriage. When I miscarried after falling pregnant by a boy I had dated for a few months right after prison, it shook me, even though I had no business having a baby with anyone else at that time in my life. I remember trying to fish the thing out of my toilet for a long time. I wanted to bury it and mourn its loss, but I couldn't get to it. It was one of those moments in my life that I replay in my head over and over: me sobbing and trying to fish something out of a toilet for some inexplicable reason. I swear death just follows me around.

There was a guy whom I dated before and after I went to prison that will always have a permanent imprint on my psyche. Now, during this time, I was using drugs. So my judgment was impaired. I also thought I was invincible. That is what drugs do to you. You forget to be scared. This guy was actually one of the nicest men I have ever been with. But he was also affiliated with one of the biggest biker gangs around. This gang rivaled the Hells Angels. I never witnessed any actual gang activity when I was dating him, but when he would take me out on his motorcycle, I noticed he would throw signs out at other bikers. We slept with a gun next to our bed. He was often in the news. Looking back, I realize it was a dangerous situation to be in. Luckily it was a short-lived relationship that just highlighted the fast and out of control life I was leading at that point in my life.

He had just gotten out of a big relationship and so had I, so we found comfort with each other. But the fact that I was on TV was obviously a huge problem for him because of his gang affiliation, and we finally ended things and both got back with our exes to try and work things out. Eventually, he died of a drug overdose like so many other people I had known. I always think about him when I am being treated badly. How is it that a man with ties to such violence can treat me nicer than a man who grew up with me and knew me better than anyone?

In addition to enjoying the company of many men over the years, I also enjoyed being with girls. When I was in drug court, I met a gorgeous girl and we started hanging out. We were both sober at the time, and we really hit it off. After a while, things just naturally turned romantic for us. We fell in love. We were a couple for eight months. I didn't really talk about it to anyone because the media was already slamming me on a pretty regular basis at this point in my life, and I didn't want to add fuel to the fire.

My relationship with that girl was deep and fulfilling. I am not at all ruling out the possibility that the true love of my life could be a woman. I felt a special closeness with her that I have yet to feel with a man, and she was more than generous and giving with her love for me. Our relationship lasted longer than my usual three-month stints and casual flings that seemed to be all of my relationships other than the big ones, and that's because she gave me everything I need from a significant other and more. However, my bad patterns were not broken yet. I still had a lot to learn about the way I act when I am in love, so unfortunately, we weren't fated to last. I still hear from this girl sometimes, and I always wonder if we could have made it if I didn't go to jail.

After a while, the girl and I fell back into drug use after we got out of drug court, and she was the one who introduced me to fentanyl. When I finally decided to opt out of drug court to go to prison, I lost touch with her, and eventually she went to jail herself. I always wonder what would have happened to us if drugs had not gotten mixed up with what we had. She was an amazing girl and I loved her deeply. I think my sexuality falls in line with my spirituality: I believe in all things and all people, just like I believe in the Universe and not one specific God. I love all people, no matter what sex they are.

My girlfriend from drug court was not the first woman I had been with in my life. I had a good friend for a while who was also a stunningly beautiful girl, and one night her boyfriend started sending me suggestive and inappropriate text messages. I told her about it, and she came over to my house to cry on my shoulder about what a douchebag her boyfriend was. One thing led to another and we had sex on the floor. It never happened again between us.

I also remember a friend a long time ago showing me how to use the new bullet vibrator she had bought. I have had some threesomes as well: overall, I think I just really appreciate the beauty of a woman's body. A particular type of woman turns me on: petite, blonde with green or blue eyes, and nice, big boobs. I would definitely say, while I prefer the company of men at this point in my life, I am, in all honesty, bisexual. Things with me are never as simple as they are for other people, and my sexuality is no exception to this rule. I just love to be in love, and I don't care what gender the person is who turns my head. I don't like boring people—that is about my only barometer for who can capture my heart.

In prison, if you got together with a girl, they called you Gay for a Day. I was kind of proud not to just be Gay for a Day. I had had a real relationship with a woman outside of jail. In jail, I had various women doing things for me like my laundry and making my food because they were romantically interested in me. I didn't fall in love in jail, however, and I really only have sex when I am filled with some sort of love for a person. I like to think I don't just get down and dirty humping and grinding. I love on someone in a passionate way. I have always been that way. I have had a lot of sex in my life, but I have also loved a lot of people.

I have had multiple ex-boyfriends contact me after we had broken up and try to solicit sex from me, or at least talk about the sex that we had as if it was some kind of life-changing experience for them. I think that is because, just like most things in my life, I give my whole self to sex with someone, and I do it in a loving way. I think giving your body to someone is the ultimate sacrifice you can make for them. And I make all kinds of sacrifices for love, for better or for worse. That is just who I am.

I have been told on many occasions that I am a natural flirt. I don't even know that I am doing it most times. I flirt with both men and women. It is just a part of who I am. When I am in a committed relationship, I like to have sex four or five times a day. I have never cheated on anyone. I have had sex in my short thirty years of life with over forty men and some women. I am certain, of course, that this is part of a mental disorder, but sometimes I think sex is a just a healthy part of life and my love of sex is an attribute, not something to be cured.

Now that I am on medication for my disorders, I have noticed my sex drive is affected a bit. Low sex drive is a side effect of antidepressants. I still really enjoy sex, of course, but it takes more work now to get me going. I think if I really examine my sexual activities closely, this might be a good thing. Over the years, I definitely have mixed up sex with love probably a little too much, and in the interest of protecting myself and my relationships, I am pretty sure this side effect of my medication is the Universe's way of slowing me down.

Obviously, my love of sex landed me on a show about teen pregnancy that pays my bills to this day, so it's hard to think of my desire for a lot of sex is a dirty secret to be kept locked up and not discussed. But clearly I needed to learn—and I am still learning—that it is possible to have too much of a good thing (even a great thing like sex).

Just after I got out of prison, a guy reached out to me online and we started to talk. He was from Canada, and he was funny and smart. We bonded over our mutual love for music and would share songs and artists with each other. We started to talk more and more. He sent me videos of himself singing Buddy Holly songs, and there was always a good morning message from him when I woke up. On my birthday, he made a cute video for me and at the end of it he said I love you. He said it in the cutest way, like he was shy to tell me. We had never met in person but over five months, we talked all the time. We had what I guess you could call virtual sex, and during those sessions he was always very considerate and caring about my needs. After a while, I realized even though we had never met, we really had fallen in love.

We talked about meeting up in Michigan, which was in between where we both lived. But before we could make a real plan, I found out the guy was married. He might even have had kids. I actually never asked. It was shattering to me. I have never been one to mess with someone's marriage, and I can't handle dishonesty in any way. Our online relationship ended before we could ever even meet in person. Over the last seven years, the guy has checked in on me periodically. I will get holiday messages from him, or a birthday greeting. I am always nice but I don't ask questions because I don't want to know the answers. It was really sad because of all the men I have been with, the one guy I never met was someone I felt one of my closest connections to. It was right when I was ending things with the married Canadian that I met someone who would take me on a three-year roller coaster ride from hell.

CHAPTER

SEVEN

The anxiety, the wait and the
complete loss of self-awareness
starts to pull over me like a dark demon
waiting for my weakest moment.
This is that day.
My weakest moment in my heart, body and soul.
I am just here.
A physical being.
Nothing I can say to help.
I am alone, even when surrounded by millions the
same.

WHEN I MET MY NEXT serious boyfriend, a short six months after I was let out of prison, I was sure this guy was going to take care of me, emotionally and financially, for the rest of my life. It began, as usual, as an online thing. We bonded over music, just like I did with the Canadian. We talked for months before we ever even met. I really liked him. He was smart and hilarious and easy to talk to. He also told me a lot of things that later turned out not to be true at all. He told me he had a million dollars in the bank, so I didn't have to worry about him being with me for my money. After months of talking, he moved to Indiana to be near me. Three months into our relationship, we were engaged.

When he moved to Indiana, I had a few of the happiest months of my life. He was so laid-back and easy to be with. Unlike my past boyfriends, he didn't need to travel to have fun. We didn't have to go out to California and hang with celebrities, or go on lavish vacations that were expensive and exhausting for me. We had fun just hanging out in Indiana, doing stuff that locals do like taking a pontoon boat out on the reservoir or hanging out at the local bars. He was very good about dealing with my extreme mood swings and learned everything he could about depression and anxiety so he could be there for me when things got rough.

I had a habit of taking my boyfriends to the local strip club, and this guy was no exception. I would throw hundred-dollar bills at the girls like I was a millionaire, and he would just laugh at my reckless spending. I could spend $4,000 a night at that strip club. I liked to think I was helping the girls pay for college. I always paid for everyone who was with us, too, and I made fun of the guys for only giving out one-dollar bills.

One night, one of the strippers invited me up on stage and I showed off my twerking skills. My fiancé just laughed and hung out at the bar with some guy friends. When a customer started talking me up, thinking I worked there, the guy I was with walked over and told him I was his fiancée. The guy who had been flirting with me stood up and we saw he was over six feet tall. My fiancé stammered, "Oh hey man, I didn't realize you were so tall! Let me buy you a drink." And I have never laughed so hard in my life. I was so happy to be with someone who was that chill and not a jealous, controlling maniac.

Around this time, my fiancé and I started a house-flipping business. I would pay for an old house in Indiana, pick out all the ways to make it special, and we would sell it for a lot more than what I bought it for. This should have been a good way for me to make six figures. This house-flipping business had the potential of giving me an extra income that might carry over when my show inevitably ended.

Another big life milestone I reached when I was with my fiancé was that I had saved up enough money to buy a house. This was a huge accomplishment for me. My daughter and I used to drive up and down the streets of my favorite suburb, Geist, Indiana, looking at all the huge houses and talking about the fact that someday we wanted to live there. My daughter was seven years old at the time, and she would say to me:

"Mommy, is this where all the rich people live?"

And I would say, "Yes, it is, and they are rich because they work hard, just like Mommy. I promise you I will buy us one of these houses one day."

And she would just give me the biggest smile.

Four years later, I did buy one of those big, beautiful houses in Geist, Indiana. I had squirreled away cash from each paycheck and put it in a little vault in my house until I had enough cash to go and buy a home. I remember going to look at my house with my friend (who was my real estate agent) and my fiancé, going upstairs to look at the master bathroom, and tearing up because the vanity in the master bath had fifteen lights. I could not believe I was going to own a house that had that many lights over the vanity. I went into the master bedroom and sat down on the bed and tears were streaming down my face. I was so happy that I could finally make good on something I had told my daughter I was going to do. I made a promise to her, and I kept it. We were going to be so happy living in that house.

After I bought the house, my daughter would come and sleep over, and we would go out during the day and do all of the family things that neighborhood was famous for. My fiancé was staying with me at that time, too, and we loved to just walk down to the water and hang out by the reservoir. He had a great relationship with my daughter and that went a long way with me. One thing I really loved about my fiancé was his ability to just hang out with me in my neighborhood, not needing to be anywhere cool or hip. Those days and the days my daughter and I spent in that house were some of the best days of my life.

Around this time, my daughter was on spring break and her dad asked if he and his wife could take her to Disney World. That would mean giving up three legally allotted days with her, but she really wanted to go, so I agreed. When she got back from that trip, I saw a huge change in her. She just seemed different and distant. She had never acted this way before, and it was so sad for me to see her pull away from me. Finally, when she stayed with me one night, I had a talk with her about it. She told me my ex had told her on the trip to Disney that I was trying to take her away from him for good.

Now, of course, I was not trying to take her away from my ex. I actually think children should spend equal time with both parents. I tried to explain this to her and tell her a little about the other things in my life that I was struggling with, but she was seven, so she could only understand so much. All she knew was the fear that was instilled in her that she might lose her dad forever, and she couldn't get that out of her head. I didn't want to force her. I didn't want her to be uncomfortable, but the whole situation broke my heart. I had finally gotten our dream house for us in a kid-friendly neighborhood that I was so excited to share with her, and suddenly it didn't seem like we were as close as we used to be. I got so depressed about it that I stayed in bed for ten days.

This was a time that my fiancé did something for me that really meant a lot. I was in a depressive state over what was happening with my daughter. He was worried about me, and he came into my bedroom and just picked me up from my bed and brought me into the bathroom. He had set up a nice bubble bath for me, and he placed me into the tub gently. It was just so nice to know that the man I had chosen to be with knew exactly what I needed on one of my low times. I took a long bath, and my depressive episode melted away with the bath bubbles. I tried to hang myself again during this time because I was so upset over the change I was seeing in my daughter, and I think the only reason I made it through this time was because he was so kind and supportive.

My fiancé and I were together for over three years. We almost eloped in Vegas. He once gave an interview in which he said that our first year together was "perfect." He got a tattoo of my name, and not a small tattoo either. Actually, my daughter's father had a six-inch tattoo of my name on him as well. He got that tattoo, incidentally, after I was arrested for kicking him down the stairs. He wanted me back and was proving his love. Come to think of it, there are in this world a total of six people who tattooed my name on them. Well, one of them died, so I guess now there are five. What can I say? For some reason, knowing me provokes some kind of need for permanence. It's kind of a nice feeling that

I can inspire such devotion, especially when I am torn apart by public perception on a daily basis.

Something held me back from actually marrying my fiancé, however, and thank God because it turned out nothing this guy told me was the truth. He did not have a million dollars in the bank. (He has some cash now, thanks to hooking up with me and booking some TV shows.) Not that I got with him because of his money. I had money of my own by then, but I was wary of guys using me for my money so it had been nice to know he had his own. In reality, he had no money and was badly in debt. The first three months we were together, he paid all of my bills like he was a Rockefeller. Turns out he was using money from his exes to pay for me.

I used to be really bad with my money. I don't live a lavish lifestyle at all, but I like to spend money on other people. When I would go out, I paid for everyone's bar tabs, no matter how many people I was with. I always want everyone to be more comfortable than I am, and my boyfriends are no exception to this rule. Back in the day, the minute I fell in love, I put whatever guy I was dating onto my bank account. Joint accounts, unchecked access to my money—it must have been fun dating me.

I once started to realize something was wrong with the way I handled my money when I went to pay for a new roof for my grandma that was going to cost $6,000, and I saw I only had $3,000 in my bank account. I didn't have credit cards, and I still don't, but I make good money. A new roof for my grandma should have been easy for me to pay for. I rarely checked my bank account balance and I had no idea where all my money went. A friend finally told me that my fiancé had a separate bank account he used to funnel money from me into. I had no idea. I never looked at my bank account balances and I trusted the men I was in love with completely.

Our house-flipping business, unfortunately for me, was completely in my fiancé's name. Although I had paid for the house we flipped, and we made a six-figure profit, I only saw $30,000 total of our house-flipping money. When I sat back and looked at the money spent and gained by that house, I realized that my fiancé had taken over $140,000 and put it in his pocket. When people ask me where all my money has gone over the years, I am embarrassed to say most of it has gone to my ex-boyfriends.

Of course, in my younger years, I blew a lot of the money I made on my show on drugs. I kept wads of cash in my house to pay drug dealers with, and my friends all knew it. There were so many times when I would notice thousands of dollars missing from under my couch cushions, and I know one of my drug-addict friends had stolen the money. For someone who seems so strong and violent, I sure let a lot of people get away with stealing from me over the years.

Once in a while, I would think about confronting someone for stealing from me, but in the end, I know it was the lifestyle I was leading that had caused the money to be gone. And I would always think that if someone took money from me, they must need it more than I did. I didn't care as much as I should have, and when it came to a guy I was dating, I cared even less. I just wanted everyone around me to be happy, and one of the things that suffered the most over the years was my bank account.

I was drinking at the time I met my fiancé, but I was trying to stay away from pills. I was doing the best I could staying away from the amount of drugs that had messed up my life so badly before jail, and my fiancé knew it was a daily struggle for me. I think the biggest red flag in our relationship was when he forced a hydrocodone in my mouth. We had just met and he wanted to see a little bit of the party girl he had read about in the tabloids. I guess depressed Amber wasn't enough for him. When I said I had given up pills, he shoved a pill down my throat. If that isn't true love, I don't know what is.

When we would fight, my fiancé would always threaten to call the police on me. I loved him for knowing everything about me and being able to push the right buttons to make me feel better when I was down, and I hated him for the same thing when things went wrong. He would throw himself down a flight of stairs during a fight and then tell me nobody would believe me if I say I didn't push him down the stairs. He once hit himself in the face and told me he was going to have me arrested for beating him. It was a bad cycle, and it only got worse. My fiancé used to slap me around on a pretty consistent basis during arguments. Never a true victim, I told him if he was going to hit me, he better kill me because I was going to come back at him tenfold. And I did.

One time, we were in Vegas filming my show when I realized I was having a miscarriage. I didn't even know I was pregnant. I was distraught. I don't do well with death, even the kind that I never knew existed in the first place. My fiancé was drunk and belligerent, and I found out he was sending pictures of our fancy hotel to his ex-girlfriends. He broke his arm that weekend and passed out from Xanax on my couch. It was my birthday. When I found a mess of loose pills in his suitcase, which he said belonged to his meth-addict son, I had to admit to myself that this relationship was in trouble. He offered some pills to my cast-mate and walked off set when he was given a lie detector test. Of course he failed the test. Nothing this guy had ever told me was the truth.

As strong as I am, however, some life events during this time took me to my knees. So even as I was figuring out that my fiancé wasn't who he said he was, I was becoming too depressed to deal with it. In addition to my many mental disorders, I also suffer from severe scoliosis. My spine curves at my neck in an alarming way. Unfortunately for me, I can't medicate for the pain caused by this because I am an opioid addict. I didn't begin using pills because of this condition, but it makes it harder for me to stay away from them. I have had chronic back pain since I was thirteen years old. That coupled with the limitations imposed on me from the combination of my mental illnesses made every day back then hard enough for me, even without the life events thrown at me that would bring a person without my demons to their knees.

About a year after I got out of prison, my dad died. I hadn't been close with him in a while, but this man was a huge presence in my life regardless of whether we were talking all the time or not. His death, even though it was the inevitable conclusion of the cirrhosis of the liver that had been eating him from the inside out for years, rocked me to my core. I can only speak from my experience, but it seems harder to lose someone with whom you have had a complicated relationship than someone who told you they love you every day. It was a huge loss for me. My dad will always be a part of my soul.

When I found out my dad was in a coma, my fiancé drove me from Indiana to Florida, where my dad lived, immediately. I stayed as long as I could but we eventually left, and as soon as I got home to Indiana, I found out he died. We turned right back around and drove back to Florida to plan a funeral with my brother. My fiancé was actually really supportive during this difficult time. He had a few nice qualities, like being good with my daughter and taking care of me when I needed help. My brother arranged a lovely funeral, and my dad was wearing an outfit I had bought him when he was buried. I didn't cry until I saw him in his coffin in that outfit. Then, standing there, I felt like all the tears I had held in for years fell from my eyes.

When my brother and I were going through my dad's things after he passed, my brother came across a few bottles of the kinds of pills that my friends and I would have loved to have in high school, the exact type of hardcore pills that had such a hold over me that I chose prison over drug court to try and conquer them. My dad was very sick toward the end of his life, and his doctors had prescribed him very strong opioids. My brother handed two full bottles of pills to me and we both just stood there. I had a moment, looking at those pills. The addict in me took a deep breath. And then I flushed them down the toilet. I wasn't completely sober, but I wasn't going to let my brother or my dad down, even though my dad was no longer here to watch me fail. It might seem like a given that one would not swallow their dead dad's pills, but I was an addict. And I was in pain. Here was one of those moments that tested me. But this time, for once, I passed.

After my dad died, things really began to fall apart with my fiancé. One thing I have learned from being on TV for twelve years is that being in the public eye, a person does not get away with lying. This guy, it turned out, had lots to lie about. I knew he had a son. I eventually met the son, who was in his twenties, and he came to live with us. My fiancé and I found the kid work on some of the properties we were trying to flip. Unfortunately, the son was a meth addict, and things did not go well with us until he finally left.

Soon, I found out my fiancé had a whole life I didn't know about: he had at least nine children with other women. He was running away from child support, and the fact that he shirked his responsibilities as a dad pretty much negated the whole reason I was still with him. We broke up but agreed to go on another reality show because the money was good, and I was probably still holding on to a scrap of hope that I was wrong and this guy was actually the answer to my prayers. He wasn't. No guy is, but it would still take me a while to learn this for myself.

I found out about my fiancé's many other kids from my daughter's father. He confronted me about it on camera. I was upset because I felt like my ex should have told me this off camera. That is how it is filming a docuseries, or what is now called a reality show, for twelve years of your life since you were seventeen years old. Nothing is private. Your best moments (the birth of my daughter) and your worst moments (there were so many) play out in a public forum.

When I was little, my dad hit me with a belt when he was angry. He also screamed at us and called me every name in the book. He was always at the bar drinking, and when he was home, he would argue with my mom. I honestly feel like I never even met my dad until he got sober when I was fifteen years old. When he was diagnosed with cirrhosis of the liver and the doctor told us he had eight months to live and my dad immediately gave up alcohol all on his own, I started to see who my dad really was. We had a lot in common, my dad and I. But they say you look for your dad in the men you date. Well, that was true, because my fiancé hit me and called me the same names that my dad did. I had found my dad in a man, just not the good parts.

Another thing my dad and I had in common that I never knew about was, as my mom later told me, that he suffered from undiagnosed depression and had even considered suicide. Even though I made peace with my dad and realized so much about why he did the things he did when I started to struggle with addiction, the framework for my issues with men was laid early on in my life. I am used to abuse and seeing fractured relationships. This is what I associated with love, and this might be why I lasted with my fiancé as long as I did.

In the times of physical abuse with my fiancé, as is usually the case with me, I have to admit the physical abuse came from both sides. The word "bitch" is a huge trigger for me because that is what my dad used to call me. My dad would yell, "Hey, Little Bitch!" at me like it was my name. When my fiancé called me that and backhanded me, I had enough of all of that, and finally one time I busted his nose. I was tired of being abused and I fought back. Like I said, I have never hit anyone who didn't hit me first.

I don't know if it was just for television or because my fiancé was so madly in love with me, but he gifted me two expensive cars—on camera—when we were together. Obviously, the $200,000 it cost to pay for these cars came from my bank account, but I still thought it was really nice of him to think of such extravagant gifts. After we broke up, I came home from a trip to California, and both cars were gone. I never saw the cars again. I thought of going to court to try and get the cars back, but I didn't exactly have the best relationship with the court at this point in my life. I chalked it up to my bad taste in men and moved on.

When that relationship ended, I still managed to mostly stay away from the pills that had almost ruined my life. I was not, however, able to handle all of the dark thoughts that filled my waking and sleeping hours. I stayed up all night watching

YouTube videos and slept late into the afternoon. I wasn't doing well. And I had not learned yet how to be quiet and at peace with being alone.

Before we parted ways forever, I agreed to film another reality show on a different network than my main show with my fiancé even though we had already officially broken up. I did it for the money, and it turned out my role on the show was basically to fight with some older ladies who thought they were good at pushing my buttons. I didn't let anyone get to me on that show; I just thought the women were pathetic. I have always had a difficult time following rules, and this show was no different. We weren't allowed to have our phones, but I had a backup phone ready to go when they confiscated mine. This should probably have been apparent to everyone as I loaded up my playlist on my backup phone and blared it in the bathroom in the morning when I got ready, but I don't think anyone working on that show noticed how much I was breaking the rules.

I wasn't very good at following directions while I filmed this show. The crew would tell me I had to be downstairs for breakfast around 8:00 AM to interact with the other housemates, and they were lucky if I appeared by 10:00 AM. I have worked for MTV since I was a child and generally followed their rules, but on this show, I felt like I was being set up to be in fights, so I rebelled a lot while filming. I did get a Mob nickname while I was filming that show. It was Pink based on the pink hair I was sporting at that time in my life. Even though I tried to tell them a famous singer already had that name, they insisted my Mob name would be Pink. So that part was cool.

The cast of this show was interesting, but I felt like because I was the only one with an active reality show at the time, I was definitely a target for the potential drama that gains ratings.

Because the other women were all older, I couldn't really connect with anyone, and one woman (a tall, long-legged giraffe of a woman) was really tasked with trying to stir up trouble with me. The burnt-out Real Housewife giraffe lady member of the cast thought it was funny to talk smack at me, and anyone who has watched my life play out on TV knows that never ends well.

One night, I was making a sandwich in the kitchen around midnight, and the Housewife's dad told me he thought maybe she was an escort. The next day, we were having a chat session, this got brought up, and I mentioned that the dad had told me he thought it was true the night before. I was just telling the truth, but it made the giraffe lady crazy. A few days later, a brawl almost broke out on the show. I took off my shoes, ready to fight. When the Housewife called me a narcissist and a victim, I threatened to flip a marble coffee table on her head. She asked me in an insulting way what the heck I was wearing, and I informed her it was an outfit from my own clothing collection that had sold out online immediately. My buttons were pushed, and I put my foot up on the table, ready to jump on her. I was ready to fight.

I wasn't scared of this bonkers lady, but I knew how to play the reality TV game, and I was ready to give the viewers what they wanted. Fortunately, security intervened and broke up the fight before it even started. Security had to stay with me overnight to make sure I wasn't going to start any trouble. My mom and I were supposed to stay in our room, but we ended up going out to make some food, and joking around with the security guards in the middle of the night. One security guard woman told me I was doing great. There was nothing but love for me from the people whose job it was to make sure I didn't kill anyone.

I actually really appreciate the quality of being a professional. I have always been a hard worker, and I have earned my own money since I was a young age. But I also feel the need to protect myself from being overly exploited, and I really felt on that particular show they were setting me up just to brawl on camera. I guess that is why I was so disrespectful on the set of that show. I was proud of myself that I did not take the bait and get arrested for assault on the set of that show, and in the end, they wanted fiery and controversial Amber Portwood to stir up things and create good television. As usual, I did not disappoint.

During my time on that show, and all the time with my fiancé, I struggled with my relationship with my daughter. I spent time with her, but I could tell she was changing her attitude toward me and it hurt. I could tell she was confused and being pulled in too many directions. Lots of times, I didn't want her around because of the violent fights I would have with my fiancé. Also, I just am not the kind of person to force myself on anyone, and unfortunately the more she pulled away, the more I let her go, hoping she would come to her senses and we could be the way we were together when she was younger.

Looking back, I realize I just didn't know how to fix what was going on with her because I had never seen a good example of how to do that. My mom and I have always been close, and we always will be. But she worked my whole childhood, so there weren't those times when we could work on anything that was wrong between us. I don't know how to sit down with a child and cultivate trust and love between us. I love my daughter like my mom had always loved me, and I always thought that would be enough. It wasn't, but again, this would take me years to realize.

Not too long after my breakup, on the set of the new reality show we were filming, I began flirting with a new boy. And my next boyfriend, once again, seemed perfect—at first. I always say you need to know someone at least a year, maybe two, before you see who they really are. It's hard to tell that to a young person, especially someone like I was back then: a person who doesn't like to listen to anyone. But it's true. All of my serious boyfriends changed a lot over the time we dated. I don't know if it was the attention they got from my show or just that I hadn't ever known them at all, but when their true selves appeared, it was a shock to me. Being on TV definitely changes a person, and you have to be a pretty strong guy to withstand the attention without letting it get to your head. You can say a lot of things about me as a person, but anybody who really knows me knows I am honest to a fault. You will know who I am within minutes of meeting me, and that does not change. I cannot say that for any of the men I dated in my younger years.

CHAPTER

EIGHT

I feel no specific emotion
At this time.
Not happiness or sadness
Triumph, even content.
Is there an emotion that is numb?
What is it called?
Is there a name?
Or am I just numb?

NOT TOO LONG AFTER I met the new guy on the set of the reality show, he moved to Indiana to be with me—and I unexpectedly got pregnant three months later. I felt guilty for having another child even though I didn't feel like I had a choice in the matter. I felt like I wasn't honoring the baby I had aborted. I had always said I would not bring another life into this world. But there he was, growing in my belly, and, just as had happened with my first pregnancy, I suddenly had the best reason in the world for staying sober.

I embraced my pregnancy as well as I could, and I kept my head above water, but I was struggling. I had gestational diabetes just like I had when I was pregnant with my daughter, and I threw up constantly and had to sleep until 1:00 PM. I was so exhausted. This added more strain on my relationship with my daughter, who didn't understand why I was sleeping so much. Without self-medicating, my internal demons got louder and louder and now hormones were raging through my system from my pregnancy. I was a ticking time bomb. Like every road I have gone down in my life, this wasn't easy and it was only going to get harder.

My son was born and, again (just like with my daughter) I was overcome with love and gratitude to the Universe for giving me this magical gift. Unlike what one might think from seeing me on TV and reading about my struggles with the law and drugs, I have always been a hands-on mom when I have the chance to spend time with my children. My daughter always looked perfect when I was with her; she was dressed nicely and her hair was always done. She always said please and thank you, and I was proud of how polite and well behaved she was.

I put my son's bassinet right next to my bed, fearful of the crib because of what had happened to my baby sister, and I got up with him countless times to feed and rock him, just like any new mom. The only difference between me and most moms was that I was still trying to find the right mixture of medications that would help pull me out of the darkness that was my life.

But even with all of my problems, and just like with my daughter, I cared for my son in the first six months of his life the best way I knew how. Then six months into my son's life, I was hit with a depression that was unlike anything I had ever felt in my life. It wasn't just depression. I wasn't just sad—I was used to that. This felt like someone came and tied heavy cement blocks onto my feet. I couldn't move. Suddenly, I was scared to hold my son. I was sluggish and lethargic all day long even though this should have been a happy time in my life. I had mood swings that did not encompass weeks or months of my life as they did during bouts of manic depression, but that changed by the minute making my outbursts and crying fits unpredictable and alarming. I had made it this far in my life dealing with mental illness but this particular type of depression brought me quite literally to my knees. It became quickly evident to me that I had postpartum depression. Add it to the list of my mental problems, for those keeping score.

When I found out I was pregnant, I stopped taking my anxiety medications because I was afraid of having a miscarriage. I had had a miscarriage in the past and had no interest in reliving that nightmare. When the happiness of giving birth to this perfect child began to subside, my old feelings of depression and anxiety came roaring back. When my son was six months old, I started having some quick blackouts and visions that I had never had before. I was lying on my bed with my son and his dad, and I had my son on my outstretched legs. Nothing stressful was occurring; it was actually a rare quiet moment for all of us. Suddenly, I had a series of really harsh and disturbing visions. That's when I started to realize something new and frightening was happening to me.

It is the most frightening thing in the world to see things that aren't there. It is so hard to tell reality from fantasy when I am having a vision. I became really scared that something was going to go wrong in real life when I was caring for my son. I hired some nannies to help me during the day, and I went to the doctor and they put me on Zoloft. But drugs like that take a while to kick in, and it turns out I didn't have any time to adjust to the medication because things went quickly downhill.

My fatigue, instability, and sudden inability to cope with motherhood came to a head six months after giving birth to my son. It was not the first time I had been arrested for domestic abuse of my partner, but it was the most widely publicized and heavily criticized incident of my life. Because of my ongoing custody battle with my son's father, I am not allowed to talk in detail about that night, but there are things that happened that are public record. The problem is, public record never tells the whole story. I have lived that hard, cold fact all of my adult life.

I always hate when people say, "History repeats itself." I feel like that is a cop-out people use to justify getting into the same mess over and over again. So I won't say that my situation that night was history repeating itself. I will say that in every situation in which I was pushed to a breaking point, I wish I had the tools and knowledge I have today. I wish I knew when to step back in those days and leave a volatile situation to deal with it in the light of day.

They locked me up that night, and after a hard three days frantically trying to get myself let out of the dreaded county jail, I was released. I could not get ahold of my partner to post my bond, and finally our house cleaner came up with the funds to get me out. The house cleaner sold some stories to the media after the event that were not true, and various nannies did as well. But I am used to being lied about, so I kept quiet about it and waited for my court date.

It is difficult not to talk about what really happened that night. I want so badly to defend myself. But it is not just the legal situation that keeps me quiet. I know I sometimes seem loud-mouthed and unfiltered, but in reality, I actually am discreet about a lot of things. I have no interest in ruining someone else's life. I have a lot of integrity, and I am not going to just run my mouth in order to make myself look better at someone else's expense.

I had been brought before the court on several occasions in my life. But this time, finally, I was well prepared. I was sober, and I had hired the best lawyers I could find: a team of super lawyers from Indiana's top law firm. These lawyers were sharp. They dressed smart, they spoke well, and they knew what they were talking about. Many of them had previously worked in the prosecutor's office so they knew exactly what was coming down the pike at me. The second we got into court and they spoke on my behalf, I breathed a sigh of relief.

Rightfully so, the judge did not send me to prison this time, but I was put on a long probation and sentenced to a batterers intervention program, as well as parenting classes. Unlike the last time I was on probation, I was determined to fulfill my probation and eager to take anything I could get out of the classes I was mandated to attend. I started to learn other ways of coping with fear and danger and intimidation through this program. Although I know this is a lifelong battle, I am hopeful my days of mug shots and court appearances are behind me for good. I was given joint legal custody of my son after that incident, the same as I was granted for my daughter. When people say my kids were taken away from me, it simply is not true. No court has ever taken a child away from me. History does not just repeat itself; things seemed to end up for me in the same way, but it was because I had work to do in my life and I was determined to do it.

When this all happened a few years ago, I reached a big turning point in my life. I had grown up witnessing violent arguments, and I never want my children to go through the same thing as me. I can't explain what used to happen to me when I was pushed to a certain degree. I saw red, and then all I would see is blackness. It is almost like I would pass out and wake up after it is all over, in shock at what had occurred. This was no way to live a life, and I was determined to find out why I acted this way and to ensure incidents of this magnitude never happened again. I am happy to say over the past two years, I have found ways to curb my anger and eliminate this violence from my life.

PART THREE
The Road to Recovery

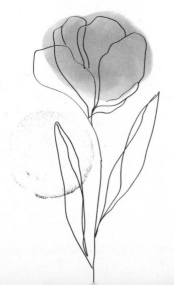

CHAPTER

NINE

Why can't they understand
The pressure, and
Force pushing down
On you?
The weight of the world
On your shoulders.
Dreadfully heavy.

THE FIRST TIME I WAS formally diagnosed with a mental illness was when I was eighteen years old. I was already on TV and had given birth to a beautiful little baby girl, but I knew something was drastically wrong with me. I had always known. I saw a doctor and was diagnosed with a severe anxiety disorder and manic depression. The minute those words came out of a doctor's mouth, I cried. My boyfriend at the time came with me and helped me understand what the words meant. I read everything ever written on the two diagnoses. Knowledge makes me feel prepared; the more I know about a subject, the more I can use this information to help myself get better. But even when I knew the facts about mental illness, I had no way to fight it. I knew what was wrong with me, but then what?

Manic depression, or what is now called bipolar disorder, is characterized by large periods of time that are filled with either depression or mania. For me, when I was not medicated, this means I would be numb and depressed for months at a time. During that time, I had no motivation to do anything except lie in bed and stare at the ceiling. I hated everything and everyone. It was an effort to brush my teeth in the morning and an effort to make coffee. When I started to feel the sadness engulfing me, I knew I had to brace myself not for hours or days of this—the sadness lasted months. There was no telling what terrible things would happen to me or what I would do to myself when I was experiencing it.

Then, when the months of depression started to lift, I would get ready for the mania. I used to live for the mania. The mania, at least in the old days, meant weeks of creative energy, marking things off of my list of things to do at a frantic pace, wild parties and late-night gab sessions with my friends, amazing sex with my partner. I was funny and smart and on top of the world. Of course, the euphoria only lasted for a short while. Then the mania would turn into a series of bad decisions, a secret or two that should not have been told, a lot of ill-advised sex, a bloody argument on a street corner, or a project begun that I could never realistically finish. In the end, neither stage of manic depression was good for me—I felt as if I was going through life like a pinball in an arcade game.

I had these mood swings for as long as I could remember. I just didn't have a name for them, and I certainly was doing nothing healthy to help stop them. Back when I was a user, I controlled my moods by using illicit drugs. I would pop a pill when I felt down and twenty pills when I was feeling dangerous and invincible. When a doctor finally diagnosed me with manic depression and having an anxiety disorder, we started experimenting with the kind of pills that are not addictive and harmful: antidepressants. Unfortunately, psychiatry and the study of mental illnesses is not an exact medical science. You don't just suture a wound and go on with your day. There is a lot of experimentation involved until the right combination of medications is obtained, and even then, there are adjustments and corrections made along the way. This is a lifelong battle.

One of the medications I was prescribed to try and help my conditions was called Abilify. I read the warnings on the side of the bottle. I was actually very cautious for a suicidal drug addict. I would often put the recreational pills I was taking into Google just to see if there was some kind of adverse effect of mixing them. Abilify seemed to have pretty harmless side effects, but it did say that there was a 5–10 percent chance of sleep paralysis. That didn't worry me; I just wanted to feel better.

Lucky me, I turned out to be in that small percentage. In the middle of the night, I woke up and could not move any of my limbs. I couldn't talk or move my mouth. I felt like some large object was pressing down on me. It happened twice in one night, and that was the end of Abilify for me. It was funny that I was taken down by one tiny little pill when I was famous among my peer group for having the highest tolerance for pills.

Back in the thick of my mental illness, I would sometimes medicate myself with marijuana. If I smoked pot, I did not need as many anxiety medications, so it helped me curb the need for the prescription drugs that had gotten me in so much trouble in my life. The legality of it is not commensurate with my current legal problems, so I don't smoke pot at the current time. However, I am a big proponent of the benefits of this particular drug.

There were many other antidepressants that I tried, and most were slightly helpful, but I didn't have that magic moment when I woke up one sunny morning feeling on top of the world. For me, these drugs made me feel slightly less depressed, but still not okay. I guess if depression was my only ailment, I might have been well a long time ago. The pills they gave me for depression were a start, but I had a long way to go.

When you begin your journey down the road to wellness as a patient of a psychiatrist, they often have you take a mental health assessment to determine your standing in the world of mental illness. It is not easy to properly diagnose mental illness. On one of these assessment tests, you are asked a series of questions, many of which are repeated in different forms to see if your answers remain consistent. This is a way to make sure you were telling the truth. In my initial mental health assessment, my answers always stayed the same, no matter how the question was asked. In this case, my brutal honesty paid off because my doctor could tell right away from my results that I was suffering from one, or maybe even two, disorders.

In the course of the next few years, I was given antidepressants and mood stabilizers, and I saw a few different psychiatrists. But to be honest, nothing was really working. I felt like my doctors just told me what I wanted to hear. Nobody was tough on me. I had not been properly diagnosed or medicated, and I was starting to make enough money to fund a pretty heavy drug habit. I look back now and realize I was lucky to make it out of this stage of my life alive.

A while before I got pregnant with my son, a lawyer in my custody case for my daughter suggested I go and speak to a psychiatrist he knew. I had seen many psychiatrists and therapists over the years. I am not an easy case. I know this. I push back and I am cynical. I used to abuse the drugs they threw at me. It is hard for me to be completely open with my doctor—mostly because I do not want to betray the trust of, or shed bad light on, all the people I love in this world. Up to this point in my life, I was convinced I could not be helped.

The minute I met him, I knew this doctor was different. He was well educated. The diplomas on his wall suggested he had gone above and beyond what had been required of him to practice his craft. He approached me differently. I respected him. He respected me. He had practical solutions to my problems, but he didn't sell me a fairy tale of recovery.

I will never forget the time I told my new doctor that my ex had made fun of him, saying he was just a kiddie doctor because he worked at Riley Children's Hospital.

The doctor laughed. He said, "I don't need to prove myself to anybody, Amber."

And right there I knew we were going to get along great. I understood that there is no cure for what I have, and I needed help to crawl out of the hole I had been in my entire life. I appreciated this doctor's brutal honesty and, at that time in my life, I was desperate to get better. Finally, I felt like I was going to get the help I needed.

At first, I didn't open up completely to this doctor. I was wary of trusting anyone at this point in my life, and I really had a hard time talking about the root of many of my problems: my family and my upbringing. I just didn't want to smear anyone's name, least of all my deceased father. But eventually I started telling my doctor some of the more painful stories of my past. After a while, he told me he thought bipolar and anxiety disorder, two conditions with which I had been diagnosed since I was eighteen years old, were only the beginning of my mental health issues. In addition to the bipolar and anxiety diagnoses, this doctor diagnosed me with borderline personality disorder. I went home and read everything I could get my hands on about this condition, and it was like he had turned a light on in my dark and muddled brain. I was finally starting to understand why I acted the way I did.

When I was diagnosed properly, my life changed. Not changed as in, "I am turning over a new leaf—this time, I really mean it!" My life changed fundamentally from the core. I was never the same again. I realized bipolar and anxiety were only the beginning of my mental issues. And that explained so much. Being bipolar can lead to long stretches of depression and mania, but why did I still snap on occasions no matter what stage of my bipolar I was in? Why did I dissociate and lose hours or days of my life? What I learned when I was diagnosed with borderline personality disorder was that I had a condition that was not only chemical, but also circumstantial. Certain triggers would set off my episodes. I learned that anything potentially tied to a trauma from my childhood would set me off. Anything that happened that triggered feelings of abandonment, anger, sadness, and betrayal—all of these things could set off a chain reaction of chemicals misfiring in my brain. When I started to realize this, the puzzle that was my brain started to feel more complete.

In addition to borderline personality disorder, after getting to know me better, my psychiatrist eventually figured out that I had post-traumatic stress disorder. I was familiar with this condition because my brother had PTSD when he got back from Iraq and Afghanistan. Every time he heard a car trunk slam, he would duck, remembering being shot at on duty. My condition was not specifically tied to one event, but to a series of events that altered my brain chemistry over the years. Seeing my dead sister, watching a man be decapitated, being called names by my dad, getting kicked out of the house by my mom, being hit with a belt at an early age—all of these early traumas combined to form this disorder. Many people with borderline personality disorder have PTSD. We are simply unable to cope with events that remind us of earlier trauma.

Now that I had a full picture of what was going on in my brain, I was able to tackle my issues head-on. Because I now knew that certain things could spark a breakdown of my defenses, I was able to know what situations to avoid. I could avoid a reaction simply by knowing that reaction was about to occur. I used my relaxation techniques and breathing exercises when I was agitated, and I just did not put myself in the way of anything that could potentially trigger me. I am still perfecting my coping strategies, and I am starting to learn how to channel these extreme emotions into more positive outlets.

I don't cry very often, but I cried pretty hard when that doctor gave me the rest of my diagnoses. I think the reason I cried so hard was because I am educated enough to know how lethal these two conditions, bipolar and borderline, are when they come in contact with each other. It's like you are about to mix up a batch of mustard gas on your kitchen counter, and the two main ingredients are inches away from each other. The combination of these chemicals can be deadly, and I knew it. With the chemicals in my brain that formulate bipolar, I am stuck in a constant vortex of depression and mania. With borderline, before I had my conditions under control, I could be subject to violent behavior that can come out of nowhere. I had no idea how I was going to manage all of these conditions. But I knew I had to try.

This newfound self-knowledge came in handy at the last reunion I filmed with MTV. At the reunion, they showed a clip that made me see red. It is always very hard for me to watch my daughter saying anything bad about me on camera. Any other season of my show, I would have lost it on the reunion stage. I probably would have clocked my ex for not defending me. Instead, I walked off the show. It may have seemed like a diva move to MTV, but I knew I was walking away from an opportunity to lose my temper. I fight every day to stay on top of my disorders, and walking off the set that day, I was just fighting again but in a different way than all of the times before.

When people accuse me of making up my disorders or using them as an excuse to behave poorly, it's hard for me not to defend myself every time I hear this or read it online. Lately, I find myself compelled to go on Instagram Live and set people straight about a lot of untrue things said about me. I try not to defend myself to the degree that I tell secrets that are not mine to keep, but I am torn apart inside by the untruths that are plastered all over online blogs. Sometimes I just have to talk about them. I am called "lazy" and "narcissistic" almost daily. I know it's because all anyone sees right now is that I am sitting on my couch. If anyone knew how hard I have to work every day between filming my show, fighting legal battles, and trying to keep my head above water, the word "lazy" would never be used in the same sentence as my name. And I am not narcissistic at all. I care more about other people than I do about myself, and that is just a fact. Again, public perception and reality are worlds apart.

Also, who in the world would want to live like a recluse, on their couch, afraid to leave their house? I wish I could be out socializing and celebrating my youth and fortunate financial situation like a normal person. When I was younger, I ignored my mental problems and tried to act like I was a typical teenager or young adult, hanging out with friends and enjoying my life. But those "normal" situations always ended badly for me, and eventually I just stopped leaving my house because I was afraid of getting into more trouble.

One of the most common traits of someone living with borderline personality disorder, and also of people living with bipolar, is that they feel things more intensely than the average person. People with either one of these disorders also act more intensely than the average person, which may explain (*explain* not *excuse*) some of the irrational, impulsive, and reckless behavior I have exhibited in the past. My fits of rage in the past could be somewhat traced to my mental illnesses. There is also history that has resulted in pent-up anger that could probably be traced back to my childhood. I don't like to make excuses, but I think it is important to realize where your behavior comes from so you can forgive yourself. So many mentally ill people are so mad at themselves for their behavior that they think they should not be alive. Forgiving yourself when you are mentally ill helps you not want to die. It is literally a survival tactic and a very important step on the way to recovery for anyone suffering from mental illness and/or addiction.

When I began seeing this new doctor, the last in a long line of doctors and therapists I had seen, he told me we were going to find the right combination of medication but that it would be a process. We started low on everything: tiny amounts of Klonopin for anxiety, small amounts of Depakote for mania and to stabilize my mood, the lowest doses possible of Clonidine and Modafinil to help regulate my sleep, and Prozac for depression. I have always known it takes more than small doses of medication to have any effect on me, but I trusted him when he told me that it was important to taper up on medications, not only to see the exact doses that work for me but also to make sure the chemicals in my brain were not altered too radically all at once.

In the past, I would take advantage of my prescriptions to fuel my drug habit. I don't do that anymore. I'm fully committed to sobriety, even if I don't participate in any of the sober people activities like AA or NA. At night I make myself my favorite cocktail, plain orange juice and cranberry, and listen to music to get a natural high instead of popping pills. I have had "sober" periods in my life before, but that usually just meant I was not terribly abusing opioids and that I still allowed myself to drink and smoke pot. These past few years I have realized that any kind of numbing is still using, plain and simple. So I let my doctor dictate the amounts of things I am allowed to take without becoming addicted, and that is all I allow myself to do. It is not easy. Fighting addiction is just as much a lifelong battle as fighting mental illness.

This doctor also stressed that medication would not solve all of my problems. He encouraged me to find other ways to stabilize my moods. Our weekly sessions were part of the hard work necessary to finally set my life on a healthy course. But when I first met this doctor, I was a complex case. I had anger issues, I had trouble integrating into normal society, I self-medicated, and I was intent on self-destruction. This doctor had his work cut out for him, and so did I.

As the doctor got to know me, he started to realize that one of my most successful coping strategies is to research thoroughly any subject that interests me. I am a voracious reader, and I have a strong interest in medicine—particularly, of course, the practice of treating mental illness. He suggested I look into a place in Indianapolis called the Indiana Medical History Museum.

He was right; I took a deep internet dive into the museum. I was fascinated. This museum sits on the grounds of the former Central Indiana Hospital for the Insane and is dedicated to memorializing and studying the beginnings of psychiatric care.

Through my research of this museum, I started looking at pictures of the ways that the mentally ill were treated over the years. I was horrified. I scrolled through pictures of skulls with holes where ice picks used to be. Sticking an ice pick into someone's brain was one of the more terrifying ways doctors tried to treat mental disorders a hundred years ago.

This hospital used to house people termed "idiots," and it was common practice to take a child with a deformity, even one as simple as a cleft palate, and put them in a crib and keep them there so long their limbs became skewed. There is a misconception that, even in the past, people who are locked up in a psych ward are sitting in a padded room with a straitjacket on, and there is a little sink and toilet, kind of like prison. The reality was actually nothing like that. There are thousands of images at this museum that feature the mentally ill pouring out of crowded institutional rooms, sitting in hallways of the hospital on the floor or in cribs, psychotic killers mixed with troubled youths, shaking and drooling all over themselves. Our country has an embarrassing and cruel history of how it treats those afflicted with mental illness.

Of course, things have slightly improved when it comes to the care of the mentally ill over the years. Nobody suffering from neuroses is strapped to a table and experimented on without anesthesia anymore. However, the stigma attached to mental illness is very much alive and well in our country. I have been told that it is not as easy for me to obtain sponsorships as it is for the other girls on MTV because of my history with mental illness. This is just a part of the obstacles I face speaking about my disorders in public. But I am determined to help other people struggling as much as I am. The discrimination and ignorance surrounding this disease of the brain is staggering.

To understand why the history of mental illness is important to me, I think it is useful to dive into my own struggles with mental illness and how my illness has affected my behavior through the years. It's funny: my mom and my brother, who know me better than anyone, have very little understanding about mental illness and how it affects the way I act. Many people think illnesses of the brain are just concoctions used to excuse bad behavior, and I know this is just because people don't understand the physiological basis for most mental illnesses. I think my most marked sign of severe mental illness is that in the past, before I got the treatment I needed, when something happened that hurt me, I didn't get sad or scared—I got angry. It is hard to have support from those you love when you act in such a self-destructive manner. And I completely understand their exhaustion.

I do not offer this analysis as an attempt to excuse my past behavior, and I have never thought of myself as a victim of any situation. But the more I learn about my conditions, the more I learn to know myself. To tell my story honestly, I have to talk about what is wrong with me. And in talking about my mental instability, I hope to shed a light on a problem that exists in our society that has always been relegated to the sidelines. Maybe if a little girl who grew up on MTV has these problems and talks about them, other little girls will come forward and get the help they need before it is too late for them.

CHAPTER

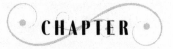

TEN

This is my time to look above even more then before
And ask for purification of my mind, body, soul
and spirit.
We ask God or the Universe for a lot.
However, if we really look closely,
He is always giving us the answers.
It is up to us, in this lifetime, to listen and search.
If we did the work, we would find that all of our
questions
Were answered.
Just within ourselves.

THE NATIONAL ALLIANCE ON MENTAL Illness (NAMI) defines bipolar disorder as: "*a mental illness that causes dramatic shifts in a person's mood, energy and ability to think clearly. People with bipolar experience high and low moods—known as mania and depression—which differ from the typical ups-and-downs most people experience. Most of the time, people in manic states are unaware of the negative consequences of their actions. With bipolar disorder, without treatment suicide is an ever-present danger because some people become suicidal even in manic states. Learning from prior episodes what kinds of behavior signals 'red flags' of manic behavior can help manage the symptoms of the illness."*

NAMI defines borderline personality disorder as this: *"borderline personality disorder is a condition characterized by difficulties regulating emotion. This means that people who experience BPD feel emotions intensely and for extended periods of time, and it is harder for them to return to a stable baseline after an emotionally triggering event. This difficulty can lead to impulsivity, poor self-image, stormy relationships and intense emotional responses to stressors. Struggling with self-regulation can also result in dangerous behaviors such as self-harm (e.g. cutting)."*

Post-traumatic stress disorder is described on the NAMI website in this way: *"Traumatic events—such as an accident, assault, military combat or natural disaster—can have lasting effects on a person's mental health. While many people will have short-term responses to life-threatening events, some will develop longer-term symptoms that can lead to a diagnosis of Posttraumatic Stress Disorder (PTSD). PTSD symptoms often co-exist with other conditions such as substance use disorders, depression and anxiety."*

And finally, NAMI lists anxiety disorders as including the following: *"Generalized anxiety disorder produces chronic, exaggerated worrying about everyday life. This worrying can consume hours each day, making it hard to concentrate or finish daily tasks. A person with GAD may become exhausted by worry and experience headaches, tension or nausea."*

Roll all of those symptoms listed above into a little ball and you might get a glimpse of what it used to be like to live an hour in my shoes before I learned how to control and manage all of my disorders. Before I had a handle on my illnesses, I might have been good TV, and a great battering ram for internet bullies back in the thick of my mental illness, but my daily battle to stay sane in the midst of all of this mental turmoil was excruciating.

Even though I have had issues with producers on my show over the years, I am grateful for the ones that protected me and took care to present me in as authentic a light as possible. Being on a reality show can be so emotionally exhausting that sometimes I wish I had ended up working in a factory this whole time, which is all I ever really expected of myself when I was younger anyway. Because I grew up so poor, however, it is just not in me to walk away voluntarily from the pile of money I earn each season. Also, I am determined to turn this platform I am given into something positive. The manic side of me threatens to quit the show all the time, but the practical side forces me to stay, earn my money, support my family, and keep my head down. I know this career won't last forever.

As I am learning more and more about my mental conditions, I am learning that my attitude toward the producers of my show kind of mirrors the attitude I bring into my romantic relationships. I build people up to this impossible standard so I can avoid any poor reflection upon myself. When they fail to meet my standards, I tear them down to devalue them and therefore preserve my own self-image. My producers are just doing their jobs. Anything bad that arises, I know, is because of the fact that I see people in absolutes and as easy as it is for me to put someone on a pedestal, it is just as easy for me to turn that person into the villain of my day. It's just a part of being me.

I can say I have come a long way in my fight against mental illness. But I still have daily struggles. Recently, I had a particularly grueling day fielding questions from producers about the status of my relationship with my daughter. The press was crucifying me once again, and internet bullies were out in full force. I wanted to stop fighting everyone: I wanted to lay down my head and rest. This is a battle I fight with myself constantly. And because I spend so much time alone, I don't really have anyone who understands how serious this is and who can talk me off the metaphorical ledge if necessary.

Even though I am on the road to finding peace and tranquility in the long run, I know any calm mental state I experience is only temporary. Years ago, when I got out of prison after serving a seventeen-month sentence, I thought I was done with drugs, done causing trouble, and I was going to take what I had learned during the CLIFF Program to help girls like me—repeat offenders who want to do better. Instead, I chased love around for a few years, had another baby out of wedlock, and got in a highly publicized fight with the baby's daddy that put me right back in county jail. The fight never ends for people like me. That is one of the hardest things to come to terms with in fighting mental illness: you are never really free.

I do, however, finally get long periods of freedom from my mental illnesses. This is just because I have been working so hard for so many years to manage them. When I am with my kids, I feel like a totally normal person. Many days now, with the right medication and weekly visits with my psychiatrist, I feel like I can conquer the world. I am a different person than I used to be, but I am wise enough to know I can never relax about my underlying issues. This is a battle I will never stop fighting and winning. I will win these fights both for myself and my children.

I have always felt a camaraderie with people in the public eye who suffer from mental illness: Britney Spears, Robin Williams, Demi Lovato, Anthony Bourdain, Chester Bennington, and others. I used to watch Robin Williams give interviews and I felt like I could see the pain in his eyes long before his mental illness was public knowledge. I knew he was masking his internal struggles with comedy even before he came out publicly and talked about it. There is something arresting about a joke told behind teary eyes. And I can spot this instantly. I have been that person, trying to be funny or smart while dying inside.

I felt a connection with Anthony Bourdain as well. I know how easy it is to mask your mental issues with drugs and how hard it is to be suffering when you are supposed to be a role model. No matter what level you are on, being in the public eye we all suffer for some of the same reasons. When everyone is watching you, it is hard not to focus on yourself. For someone with depression, that focus is going to be negative. It is inescapable, no matter what situation you are in.

The situation with Britney Spears hits close to home as well. She most likely had these chemicals misfiring in her brain from childhood. And the scrutiny of the public just magnified everything until she went completely crazy. I can relate. When news of my first arrest hit the airwaves, the press would not leave me alone. And I was drowning in pill abuse and suffering from multiple mental disorders. The magnifying glass you are under when you are the focus of the press is oppressive and can make your mental state worse. Britney has been very open about not being able to handle her own finances or have custody of her children, and I appreciate her honesty and hope this helps shed light on the mental health community just like I am trying to do. At the very least, maybe online bullies will stop picking on people like us and realize that there is something very serious going on with someone who is so obviously troubled.

When a celebrity commits suicide, it is difficult for the public to understand. Growing up as poor as I did, it always felt to me like money would definitely make things better. Well, I am living proof that money does not solve your problems. Money and fame actually can make things worse for a clinically depressed person. There is more pressure on you when you are watched constantly and when you mess up, and you will, the criticisms are loud and unending. Also, when you are mentally unstable and using drugs, it is hard to make sound financial decisions. As a celebrity, there is pressure to look good and to say the right thing, to never fail. On top of that the intense scrutiny of my parenting being on a show about being a teenaged parent—which combines notoriety with the most personal job a woman can have, being a mother—this is a recipe for a mental health disaster.

I have clearly survived years of online bullying, and likely even come out stronger for having had to deal with it. But I worry about people who are not as strong as I am. If I am getting pummeled for what seems like a rant on Snapchat or Instagram Live that was instigated by watching my ex lie about me on my TV show, I wonder about the other ex-drug addict, ex-con moms out there who are fighting to keep their heads above water. An attack on one of us seems like an attack on all of us, and I think that has to stop.

According to the National Institute of Mental Health, suicide is the second leading cause of death for people ages ten to thirty-five. Also, according to CNN, the highest suicide rates for women are in the fields of arts and entertainment. I know why this is the case. The pressure on women in our society today is immense—add to that the magnifying glass of social media, and it is overwhelming. I feel pressure every day. My days are filled with paperwork for court dates, writing assignments for my probation officer, calls with agents and my manager trying to figure out how I am going to make a living once my tenure on MTV is over, and my lawyers figuring out a way to see my children more. I have a bad habit of unleashing my frustration—especially on a week my show airs—on Instagram Live, and the next day is spent fielding insults from fans that were offended or frantic calls from my team. My relationship with Instagram Live is complicated because on the one hand, it is sometimes the only contact I have with the outside world. And it is therapeutic for me to be able to use that platform; however, I know I can come across a little unfiltered and raw, and I am working on that.

I am a strong person. But people need to know that there is violence in their words online. When I read comments on my Instagram saying that I am a waste of space, these are words that feel like a physical blow to me. And I know people with mental disorders who follow me feel that blow themselves. *If Amber doesn't deserve to live, what about me?* they think to themselves. They read the comments and realize they have been away from their kids and in jail for years, so *if Amber is a bad mom, I must be ten times worse.* And then I wonder if anyone who follows me because they suffer from one or more of the same mental conditions I do has turned around and committed suicide. We would never know why this happened, or that it happened at all, but the power of destructive words on the internet cannot be underestimated. Trust me, I know.

There is a well-known quote about fame and what it can do to a person's psyche:

> *"In the urge to find a better, more perfect self, the possibility of uncovering a worse, more misshapen one hangs like a threatening cloud. Lurking behind*

every chance to be made whole by fame is the axeman of further dismemberment."

Leo Braudy wrote this in his book *The Frenzy of Renown*. This could not be truer when it comes to me. Here I am, trying everything I can to overcome my illnesses and clean up a debilitating drug habit, and I have to watch my daughter talk about how we don't get along on TV every week. I have to read endless comments about how I am a terrible mom, a waste of a human, and a person who does not learn from her mistakes and take any accountability for her actions. Being famous and on TV is not as fun as it looks.

Whenever I read about a celebrity or an influencer committing suicide, I know that in the past, before I got the treatment I needed, that it could have been me. I can picture the covers of the magazines if one of my suicide attempts had actually succeeded, and I can hear the comments on my Instagram page in my head. Of course, people will say what a cop-out it was, how I was abandoning my children, and how ungrateful I was for the things fame and money have allowed me. But in reality, even a strong, resilient girl like me has to give up fighting at some point. I feel much better lately, and I am a fighter. I just worry about people who cannot weather the storm of mental illness as well as I have.

#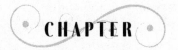

ELEVEN

Isn't Monday the worst?
People say.
That's when everyone is working.
Weekends are gone.
The fun is over.
The sleep and rest is not allowed.
But, then, what about Tuesday?
Oh I dread this the most.
I die a little on Tuesday
Just to be numb.
It helps the pain.
See, I dread Tuesday, not Monday.

I USED TO WAKE UP SOME mornings and the first thing I saw is myself hanging from my ceiling fan. It was a pale, dull fan that creaked ever so slightly as it spun. I would look up in a haze of sleep medication and there I was with dead eyes, spinning around, bound by some kind of rope. I don't know why, but in real life hanging was always my preferred method of self-annihilation. So maybe that's why I used to see myself hanging above my bed sometimes in the morning when I woke up. Or maybe it's because I really was crazy just like everyone said.

When things were really bad for me, sometimes I would be making myself a sandwich during the day and I would have a brief glance of myself cutting my own throat with the butter knife I was using to spread mayonnaise on the bread. I would black out for a few seconds and wake up and go on making my sandwich. Once in a while, I would be putting on makeup and suddenly I would see an image of myself punching the mirror. My wrists were cut and there was blood everywhere. Then the flash would end and I would go back to putting on my makeup. I have real-life marks on my neck where I have brought a knife with the intention of slitting my throat. I have scars on my body from cutting myself for years. And I used to have visions of my own death all the time. These bouts of psychosis were frightening and debilitating. Although I would love to have full custody of my children, and even though these visions have subsided in the past few years, the fact that I ever even had these psychotic breaks might mean that will never happen. It's something I have to learn to accept as part of having these illnesses.

I lost three days once. I was sitting on my couch on a Monday. I had not been diagnosed properly and had not received treatment for my illnesses. I didn't remember a thing. And when I came to, it was Wednesday. I was wearing the same clothes. My hair was a little messier. I had no idea where the three days went. Sometimes the blackness was fleeting, and sometimes it would go on for hours or days. There was no way to really know what happened during these episodes, especially the ones that happened since I started living alone. This happened when I was abusing drugs and when I was not. These blackouts, whatever their duration, were just a part of my life before I got things under control.

I've learned how to overcome the blackouts. They were more frequent and intense when I was under an unusual amount of stress. But now that I have undergone treatment and am medicated properly, they do not happen anymore. To begin to conquer them, I tried meditating. I spoke out loud to the Universe. I read books. I wrote. I lay down and rested. I had no choice but to cope, especially when my self-medicating days were over. I have become spiritual, but not in any defined or organized way. I believe in life and death, and everything in between, every religion and no religion. I love to read about philosophy. Epictetus, Socrates, and Aristotle. My living room is adorned with books by everyone from Einstein to Sun Tzu. This is how I get through my minutes, absorbing the words of others to quiet the voices in my head.

Over the past twelve years, since I started my journey as a reality television personality, I have been contacted by thousands of people who are, or think they are, suffering from the same mental illnesses as I am. To be honest, I am always skeptical of other people's versions of what I have. Sure, you might be bipolar. Or you might have borderline personality. But take both of those conditions, throw in a large dose of anxiety and PTSD, and then you really might know how hard things were for me at one point in my life. I am envious of people who, for example, go through a breakup and suffer from depression. They go to a doctor, get put on antidepressants, and voila, they feel better in six months. That is not my experience with mental illness at all. What I have will never go away, but thankfully it can be regulated with therapy and the right medication. What I have I did not cause, and I do not perpetuate by my actions. It is a part of me, it is something that I have to be aware of every day, and it will always be that way.

One of the byproducts of my illnesses is the fact that I used to experience episodes of psychosis. I don't have these episodes anymore, but I want people to know what having my mix of mental illnesses before I got it under control was like. Here is an example of a psychosis: before I was properly diagnosed and medicated, a fan on my social media would reach out to me. They were angry with me for something they saw on my show, or maybe it made them feel good to pick on an easy target. They would tell me to slit my wrists and watch the blood drip down the side of my bathtub. Hours, or a few days later, I was in the bath. Suddenly I saw, as plain as day, blood pouring out of my wrists, down the side of my bathtub, and all over my bathroom floor. Seconds later, I blinked and it was gone. This used to happen to me all the time: I would see glimpses of things that were not there. It is a difficult way to live, and sometimes I have no idea how I got through those days.

Even to this day, it is difficult for me to film my TV show outside my home because of my anxiety. I don't like talking about my personal life where other people can hear me. It makes me feel like I am going to have a panic attack. That sounds crazy coming from someone whose job it is to participate in entertaining television. I have taken a beating from people who view the show for not moving around a lot when we film, but there is a reason I am most comfortable in the safety of my home and the comfort of my couch. In the outside world, though, fans don't understand why I don't go anywhere, and fans can be my saving grace or relentless in their attacks on me.

Recently, I was at a restaurant filming with my mom. My mom was crying. A waitress remarked that she was a big fan of mine. Later that day, she, along with some other restaurant staff members, posted on social media that I was at their restaurant and my mom was faking her tears. They made fun of me. The internet had a field day. There goes Amber again, faking drama, her mom with those crocodile tears! This is why I rarely leave my house. This is how mental illness combined with fame affects my life.

One thing I have learned from years of psychoactive medication is that nothing works all on its own, and you are never okay forever. Even if what you are doing works for a while, your problems might rear their ugly heads anyway. I am sick for life. Nothing truly takes these dark feelings away, at least not for me. There is no magic pill that cures bipolar or borderline personality disorder. Actually, there might be pills that cure mental illness that exist but "Big Pharma" certainly is not going to introduce them to the market and take away the cash cow that is the pharmaceutical drug trade.

What helped me conquer the demons that used to plague my life was a combination of regular visits with a good and caring psychiatrist, the right combination of medications, and learning ways to recognize signs that I wasn't feeling quite right so that we could adjust what I was doing or taking before things got bad. It took me a while to get to this place in life, but I can honestly say I have figured out how to function normally. It is a great feeling after so many years of darkness.

There are some good pills out there that help with anxiety, but unfortunately, they are also very addicting. The right non-addictive medications, education, coping methods, relaxation techniques, and intense psychoanalysis—all of these combined might help me start to gather the tools necessary to get through any given day. But every day is different, and my triggers are everywhere. The hallucinations that used to be a part of my daily struggle in the thick of my mental illness days can be eliminated by intensive therapy and proper medication. And thank goodness, because it is a scary thing to not know if what you are seeing in front of your eyes is real or not.

What has helped me tremendously in getting a handle on my disorders is therapy. Something interesting I have learned after more than three years of intensive psychotherapy is that people with borderline personality disorder often use important people in their lives for replacements for how we see ourselves. For example, my psychiatrist says I used to use the men in my life to see myself in a better light. If I think my boyfriend is perfect and he loves me, well, I must be perfect too. It's a way I learned to build myself up because I had been beaten down so much of my childhood. I had never thought of love this way: I am a romantic at heart, but a lot of what I learned fit perfectly into my usual pattern of falling in love.

It turns out, my psychiatrist tells me, that if my significant other disappoints me, they lose their value in helping to boost my self-esteem. People with borderline personality disorder sometimes do something called "splitting objects" into good and bad. When a good object fails me, my rage at the disappointment and sense of shame this makes me feel causes the object to become completely bad in my eyes. In real life, to normal people, everyone is a combination of good and bad. But to someone with my condition, people are either just good or bad. That is how I got through my childhood, being able to put good and bad in different categories so I could understand them better and tackle them easier.

Turns out, my need to split people into two parts, the good and the bad, stems from the abuse I suffered as a child. When my dad, whom I needed as a protector and nurturer, called me horrible names, I separated that side of him from the side that was my loving and caring father. That way I could hate the bad side of him but still depend on the good side as I grew and needed support. When children of abuse grow older, they can bring this survival technique into their adult life. I love my boyfriends fiercely until I hate them ferociously. It's a destructive cycle that I had to work to break. To stop seeing people in extremes, I had to learn to accept myself in a way that was healthy and realistic. The amount of work that required was staggering, but I can say I no longer see people in such extremes.

I guess a simpler way of putting it is that my relationships ended so often and sometimes so quickly because I put my boyfriends on pedestals that they were going to fall off of. I had to learn that disappointment is inevitable. I have realized that nobody is perfect, no matter what superficial things point to perfection. I have noticed in my life that most of my relationships, besides my three long-term ones, have lasted an average of about three months. That's because it took a few months for me to realize there is something wrong with whomever I am dating. It never occurred to me that there is something wrong with everyone, and nobody is as bad as the worst day they have ever had. I should know that better than anyone, I guess.

It turns out my expectations in a relationship were beyond impossible to fill. I also always ignored big red flags in a relationship, and I guess in retrospect that was because I was so busy building this random guy into my perfect soul mate, I lost track of all of the signs pointing toward the dangers ahead. I am trying now just to take things ridiculously slow when I date. The stakes are too high for me to get involved in a bad situation once again. I have also noticed that some of my habits when it came to relationships just aren't there when it comes to dealing with my children. I have a much healthier outlook as a mom than I did as a girlfriend. I am thankful I somehow learned from a young age how to love your children completely without conditions or unrealistic expectations.

As I delve into my romantic relationships in therapy, I see that when these "perfect" men failed me and turned out not to be perfect, it was my dad all over again, disappointing me and hurting me. I tore these men apart, physically and emotionally, for being flawed as a way to not have to face what was wrong with me. If the man was worthless, well then, I was still perfect because I had no part in their failing. It was a very serious cycle of self-protection and anybody who stood in the way of this was in the path of a cyclone.

A good example of not recognizing serious red flags in a relationship might be ignoring the drug use of my partners. It's no secret I had drug addiction problems. Regardless of this, I used to fall into men who did drugs. I used to be attracted to that fast way of life and to men who are broken in some way. I definitely used to be the kind of person who likes to help the wounded, and drug addiction was just another wound I thought I could help someone heal. I have finally realized that if I want to live a happy and healthy life, I just can't involve myself with anyone who uses drugs. All of these realizations have helped me see the patterns in my love life and try my hardest not to repeat them.

I truly feel now that I could be in a healthy and sustained romantic relationship. But I am done with bringing a series of different men around my children, and I cannot afford to have anyone else take advantage of me as my career shifts and I get older. I never wanted to be one of those teen moms with multiple baby daddies. It actually embarrasses me that I have two of these, and I have no intention of adding to that list. That being said, however, I like being in love, but I can say now that finding a partner is not my main goal in life.

CHAPTER

TWELVE

Waking up every morning
With pain within my body,
This is my time for renewing
Accepting and completing
This chapter of my life.
This is my time to look above
Even more than before
And ask for purification
Of my mind, body, soul, and spirit.

O NE QUALITY THAT ALSO SEEMS to be common in people
with borderline personality disorder is that people with
this condition tend to get into a lot of heated arguments and
physical altercations. I used to get into fights on a regular basis
pretty much anywhere I happened to go. I guess a combination
of being a master number eleven and a Taurus, coupled with
neurons firing at record speed in my head and the fact that I was
a local celebrity who had aired a lot of dirty laundry on television,

was the perfect recipe for public discord. This is something I have worked hard in therapy to overcome, and I am proud to say I am a different person now when it comes to resolving conflict.

I think the most publicized public brawl I ever had happened at a breakfast place in Indiana. This was years ago, before I figured out why I was acting that way and how to stop it. It is a good example of how I used to act and how far I have come, as nothing like this has happened in years. I was with an ex, a really sweet guy but one of those three-months-and-out types, having a post-bar bite to eat when I heard a girl sitting at the table across from us mention my name. I distinctly heard her call me white trash. When the words "bad mom" came out of her mouth, I rose up. I try to tell people this all the time, and it's not my fault if they don't listen: you really do not want to mess with me.

I listened to this girl trash-talk me, and I slowly took off my jewelry. I was ready to fight. Now, I don't necessarily think this is something to brag about, but you really don't want to fight me. Back then, I had not begun any formal kind of fight training. All I saw is red when I was provoked. I also did not care about anyone in the world besides my family. I would bash someone's head into the ground over and over until I saw blood pouring out of them. And this girl would not stop talking. She just sat at her table, running her mouth, and at first, I just told her to shut up. Any smart person who knew anything would have paid their check and gotten out of there, but this girl had something to say. So I got up from my table and approached her.

The girl did not get up from her seat, nor did she shut her mouth. I pushed a coffee pot off a counter toward her. She jumped up and grabbed at my hair and tried to hit me with a sideways jab. Trying to defend myself, I took hold of her wig as she swung at me and held onto my hair, and started punching her in the face with uppercuts. Her wig came off, and I sent it flying across the restaurant. The manager called the cops, and the fight was broken up in minutes. To her credit, this girl did not press charges or get the police involved herself. She even asked me less than politely to finish the fight with her in the parking lot. I just laughed and left. This girl had no idea what a monster she was unleashing. It was for her own good I did not take her up on her offer.

Of course, pictures of the fight hit the press almost immediately. I have had my share of legal troubles, but so far, I have never gotten arrested at the scene of a fight. Partly, I suppose, because it was always immediately apparent that the other person had instigated the fight, and partly because I knew most of the owners of the establishments in which the brawls took place. Regardless of the reason, it is remarkable to me that this chapter of my life has avoided the long arm of the law.

I've never been badly injured in a fight, but a girl who would not stop haranguing me for being on television ("I was a pregnant teen and I didn't get no TV show!") pulled on one of my feather earrings once. It left my earring hole permanently elongated through the bottom part of my ear. It's good to have that reminder of the beast I used to be. I had an imprint of her tooth on my knuckle that lasted a few weeks, and it was a slight indicator of the way that fight could have turned out. Most of the fights I have been in are a blur to me, either from all the pills I had taken or because of the hefty adrenaline rush that accompanied each one. Being in fights is not something I am proud of, and it took years for me to figure out ways to avoid them.

I discovered mixed martial arts about ten years ago. I was getting into fights pretty regularly by then, especially as my TV show gained popularity. Back then, I just could not ignore all of the comments I heard from jealous girls in a crowded bar and felt the need at the time to approach anyone talking smack about me and invite them to repeat their rude comments to my face. I was smart enough to know that if I did not strike first, I might not be arrested, but it was never hard to entice some trash-talking female into taking a swipe at me. I was not a trained fighter, but I was scrappy and tough, and as long as someone didn't have my hair wrapped up, I could give a good beating to pretty much anyone.

As my show got more popular, the trash talking got meaner—and the pent-up aggression I felt from years of being screamed at as a child started to grow. I found myself not able to stop smashing someone's head into the ground. I would punch girls' heads into the ground until I saw blood and then keep going. I had an easy on switch, and apparently no off switch when it came to fighting. Finally, I knew I needed another outlet for my anger. That, and also because I wanted to keep winning these fights and not end up in a hospital, made me look into practicing mixed martial arts.

What made me take up martial arts and continue it to this day is that it is a way for me to channel my aggression. It is funny to think that learning to fight is a way to keep myself from fighting, but it's true. Studying martial arts is one of the ways I control my mental illness. It is rewarding and therapeutic and helps me become my best self: a peaceful warrior.

When I began, I started taking classes in Krav Maga, or Israeli jujitsu. I had sparring matches, mostly with boys. I was terrible at first, but I got better and was able to hold my own. I loved learning to control the powerful jabs and kicks associated with this addicting way of fighting. But it was the melding of mind and body that came with karate that really took my heart, and once I started practicing this art form, I knew I had found something that would follow me for the rest of my life.

Karate was immediately appealing to me because it actually does not just teach you how to fight well. More important than fighting, karate teaches you restraint, and up to this point, in almost every aspect of my life, restraint was something that was far out of my reach. Karate also helps you stay humble, and that is something that is important to me in all aspects of my life. Karate helps me calm the voices in my head, and has helped me gain awareness of where my real strength lies. I learned through karate that it doesn't make you strong to confront a loudmouthed girl in a bar; it makes you strong to walk away from that girl. I hope I never stop practicing karate because it has become something that has added so much light to my life. My sensei has become an important mentor to me. I work with him almost every week, and he helps me learn the skills necessary to advance through the belt system.

I think another benefit for me of doing karate is that I am proud of how good I am at it. Karate is not easy; there are complicated moves to learn, and to go through the belt system takes discipline and skill. I am aware of the negative public perception I hold because I was a drug addict and I have been to jail. Back in the olden days, if someone acted the way I did, society would say I had "brought shame upon my family." My actions have always brought on an especially public and hurtful assault from the media and internet bullies, and as strong as I seem on the outside, the blows strike deep, especially those directed toward my physical appearance and my parenting skills. When I got good at martial arts, I became more peaceful, and the hurtful comments from the outside had less effect on my inside than they used to.

Another thing that has helped me fight the aggression and mental illness is meditation. I have my own method of meditating that I learned from watching YouTube videos during sleepless nights, and some of it I made up on my own. It is something I practice many times a day. I begin by holding my breath for ten seconds, and then I increase that until I reach almost a minute of holding my breath. This helps clear my mind from chatter, helps ground me when I am feeling unstable, and gives me the clarity I need to deal with the myriad situations that give me stress and anxiety. Holding my breath and clearing my mind can sometimes feel as good as doing drugs back in the day. Karate and meditation, along with reading, have kept me safe and harmless for the past few years.

I know I was born a fighter. I come from a whole family of fighters. My mom had to wear braces on her legs when she was little, and she was deaf in one ear and blind in one eye. She worked so hard my entire life at job after job, fighting to take care of my brother and me even while she was in pain. When I was little, she worked nights and my dad was the one who braided my hair and took me to school. My brother enlisted in the Army when he was in high school and served in Iraq and Afghanistan. My dad fought liver disease for years beyond what the doctors thought was possible. We are not people to shy away from an argument or a challenge: we are an assertive and fearless family. When my mom was little, she had to find food in dumpsters and didn't even have a bathroom; they had to pee outside. Her family did not have utilities for ten years when she was growing up. Poverty can instill a kind of strength in you that people who grew up comfortably will never know. I come from a family of hard workers, and my commitment to mixed martial arts and karate feels natural to me because strength and fighting is in my blood.

There are good and bad kinds of fighting, I have learned. Kicking your boyfriend in the back so he falls down the stairs or hitting your partner because you are mad at him or he hit you first are both the bad kinds of fighting. Winning a sparring match with a girl twice my size in a ring, however, is a good kind of fighting. I am proud of the fact that this kind of fighting is still in my life and, hopefully, the other kind of fighting is done for good.

CHAPTER

THIRTEEN

I look around and feel safe and trapped.
I feel a cage holding a bird,
Perhaps a vulture?
It attacks with such force it scares its prey,
The same animal that shot it down.
Bullets, or words, or stones or just a poke.
Enough to provoke its inner power, its soul of
wisdom
Is noticed after but not before.
There's no sleep for the owl, however the prey sleeps
at night,
My time of wisdom, education, and eventually a
tactical attack!

THE MEDIA HAS BEEN A villain in my life since I was seventeen years old. But the media is not some evil person I can just give a roundhouse kick to and walk away. The media is a whole network of people who are tasked with taking people like me down for a living. There is no way to fight the media, and I feel helpless even trying. It is crazy to me that online publications can say anything they want and there is no recourse to fight them. Of course, if you are Tom Cruise, you can spend millions to rehab your image, but I am not Tom Cruise. I have to live with the fact that lies are printed about me every day.

I take full responsibility for the real actions that placed me in the headlines, but the media definitely takes coverage of my behavior too far. The media has been generating ugly headlines about things that have happened to me since before I was even a full-grown adult and able to process what they were saying about me. I can be called fat and lazy and a bad parent on any given day, even on those days when I am doing well in all of those areas of my life. The truth does not seem to matter as long as the headline entices people to read.

I am aware that over the years I have given the media plenty of material for attention-grabbing stories. I have been to jail five times. I have been pregnant multiple times. I have had two babies, both at a very young age. I have gotten in public fights, I have ranted on social media, and I have called my exes horrible names. I have even called out my fans and threatened to fight them. I have given everyone lots to talk about and I understand that comes with the territory. That's not what gets me. Cover what I have done, sure. I am used to it after years in the public eye. But editorializing as part of reporting is a more recent phenomenon and with that, I feel powerless.

When the media attacks me, it reminds me of the bullies that I knew in my high school in Anderson, Indiana. The articles they print about me sometimes remind me of a note I might have gotten from the school bully. The note would have been misspelled and the grammar would probably have been wrong, and it may have seemed like they were talking about somebody else. A bully might call me a pig or white trash, and I honestly had no idea where they got those impressions of me. The person the media has created to gain clicks and sell magazines also, to me, has nothing to do with who I am in real life.

Over the years, I have kind of accepted my role as the "bad mom" and "drug addict" on my show, but when article after article, year after year repeats falsehoods, it wears on me. Wikipedia, for example, is a supposed online encyclopedia of fact, and I even paid them $1,000 one time to make sure their accounting of my life was accurate. What they have listed on there now has many mistakes. I have never possessed crack or meth, and the fact that criminal is in the first sentence of my bio there feels sensationalist and mean. Most of the facts of my life are either televised or recounted in public court records, so it makes no sense that this online encyclopedia would get facts wrong. It's not that hard to get it right.

I remember when my brother and I were going through my dad's things after he passed away. I was so surprised to see that my dad had collected every single magazine in which I appeared. Didn't matter if the story was good or bad, my dad held onto it. One magazine even printed: "Amber Portwood is a Monster!" on its cover, and my dad had that issue in his stack of other magazines. I'm not a monster, of course, and it makes me sad that my dad, who was so sick for as long as I can remember, not only had to read that about his daughter, but he kept it as a souvenir all these years.

What upsets me the most about media bullying are two things: one, I was a child when it all began. Who picks on a child? Specifically, who picks on a child who is just becoming a mom and who is new to the game of branding and creating a character for television? I was a kid, just being me, and I was made to be a bad guy from the very beginning. I don't mind if the facts are reported. I am happy to help sell magazines, but I hate when they get the story wrong and paint me out to be something I am not. And it has gotten far worse in recent years because there aren't enough scandalous real events for the reporters to write about. So they make stuff up.

Another thing that bothers me about the way the media has sometimes treated me is that it is public knowledge that I suffer from mental illness. My suicide attempts and my stay in a psychiatric ward have also been part of the public record. I wonder about the conscience of a person who makes fun of a girl who has the issues I have had. I am a strong girl. I can take the abuse and come back even stronger. But I worry that if I do not speak up when I am mistreated, misquoted, or just lied about, I am not standing up for my community of mentally ill people who are similarly chastised for their conditions.

Today, hiding from the press has become just like hiding in the bathroom stall for forty-five minutes during lunch period in high school so I didn't have to face the kids in my school who made fun of me because my boyfriend dumped me. The only difference between now and then is that back then, I would find a pill to swallow that made all the pain go away. Now, I just have myself to lean on to try and make sense of all the meanness in the world. I always dream that one of these days, the mentally ill will band together and rise up. If we ever can gather our forces and stamp out the bigotry and ignorance that is thrust upon us so cruelly, God help you all.

I somehow survive the constant barrage of insults from the online community and I think it is because, in the end, I try and not absorb the bad things they are saying about me. I go forward because I believe in myself and because, deep down, I know the awful things they are saying are just not true. The people who love me know I would do anything for them. When I have set out to achieve something in life, I have usually accomplished the goal. I am an advocate and educator when it comes to my struggles, and I will continue to be vocal about these things, no matter what everyone says about me.

I have never lied about the bad things I have done. I am open about my shortcomings, and I am aware my pill abuse and aggression were problems that needed to be addressed head-on and not swept under a blanket of diagnoses. Just like being provoked does not excuse hitting someone in the face, having a violent argument in front of your child is wrong no matter what your psychological makeup says about you. But being mentally ill is a part of who I am and is a part of what I do. It's not an excuse; it just is part of the reason why.

I am so vocal about mental illness because I want to use the platform I have been given by MTV to raise awareness about the illnesses that have killed millions of people. I don't want to see those who are not as strong as me cave under negative scrutiny and bullying and die by suicide. I realize emphasizing this subject so forcefully opens me up to the criticism that I am using it as an excuse or to whine about what a victim I am. I am not. I am writing about my diagnoses and what has helped me so that I might reach those that have had the same issues as me in an attempt to destigmatize mental illness. Perhaps hearing my story might make some people less afraid to speak up about mental illness and get the help they need. At least that is my hope.

FOURTEEN

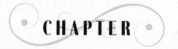

I still see myself from the outside,
Like a movie.
I look very peaceful.
I know this won't last long.
Eventually my image is gone
And I hear good morning again.
Maybe tomorrow
I'll dream differently.

I HAVE NEVER REALLY WARMED UP to Alcoholics Anonymous or Narcotics Anonymous. I have attended meetings but nothing said in those meetings really helped me. I am generally not a joiner anyway. I prefer to self-educate and learn things the hard way. I have no idea how many days I have been sober; I haven't kept track and I like to live life day by day anyway. It has definitely been a few years since I have abused prescription medication or drank alcohol. That is not to say, however, that I am my own lucid, intelligent, well-read self every day of the week.

The constantly adjusting chemicals in my brain rule my moods so I have to deal with the properties of mental illness just like I used to have to live with the effects of abusing pills.

Last summer, my sobriety was tested once again by the death of my beloved grandma. Her death was sudden and a complete shock to me. She had stage four pancreatic cancer, something none of us knew until it was too late. That woman had been living with cancer and never even knew it; that is what a badass she was. Anyone who knew my grandma loved her, and I loved her the most of all. Before I was even on TV, my grandma was my biggest fan, and her unwavering support was always a beacon I could go to in any storm, and I feel rudderless and alone now that she is gone.

My grandma was the OG badass. She taught me to face adversity with bravery and never to shy away from conflict. She was a lunch lady at a school for thirty years, so I clearly got my work ethic and humility from her. Every time in my life that I have felt like curling up into a little ball and hiding from the world, grandma was the one who encouraged me to not only look life in the eye but shine through it. There is nothing to be embarrassed about being cursed with the diseases of mental illness and addiction, and I can thank my grandma for instilling in me the pride that carries me through most events in my life. There are only two people left in this world, besides my children, who mean as much to me as my grandma: my mom and my brother. If something happens to them, I would be devastated.

Another event that happened to me in the past year was the death of my dog, Madison. Madison was with me for years and was the only thing standing between me and complete isolation and solitude. When my dog got sick, I missed parenting time with my son. Although I never want to do anything to compromise what little time I do spend with my son, I will defend my decision to take care of my dying animal and not wanting to expose my young son to the horrors of death as I was exposed to them at such a young age. The loss of a pet is hard on everyone, but for someone who feels like every day is a new nightmare of survival, the death of a long-time friend such as Madison was a crushing blow.

When things like my grandma's death and the loss of my dog happen to me, I have to suddenly pivot and find ways to prevent these events from affecting my mental health and my sobriety. I love to read. I read a lot. I read Latin books to my son. I love philosophy and reading about the Greek men who shaped our society today.

Epictetus is my favorite philosopher. That man was a crippled slave; he had nothing going for him at all, yet he was filled with wisdom that made him memorable. Epictetus taught that we need to accept things that happen to us calmly, and that we are all responsible for our own actions and must use self-discipline to conquer adversity. He was all about honesty and self-education, two things that are very important to me. It is through learning about different philosophers that I have found ways to cope with some of the more heart-wrenching things that have happened in my life.

Epictetus says that when you lose someone you loved, you should say to yourself, "I have lost nothing that belongs to me; it was not something of mine that was torn from me, but something that was not in my power has left me." He talks a lot about things we can and cannot control in our lives and how to handle both of these instances gracefully. His writings are very forgiving of poor behavior, and I find that comforting as I examine the wrongs I have committed in my life. Epictetus says, "Those who go wrong we should pardon and treat with compassion, since it is from ignorance that they err, being as it were, blind." I have been figuratively blind for a lot of my life, so I can really relate to quotes like these.

Socrates also talked about ignorance and how this is the one true evil in the world. I confess to being ignorant at times in my life, and I am still learning. I definitely feel like I can see ignorance around me a lot. People are ignorant about the mentally ill. They are ignorant about opioid addiction. Ignorance is everywhere. I also like the way Plato talks about the world in that he reminds us the difference between speaking just to hear oneself talk and actually being wise for saying something with meaning. I have found comfort in learning from these important contributors to a civil society, and I really think this appreciation for their wisdom has helped me navigate the rough waters that have so often disrupted my life.

Along with studying philosophy, I like to read writing that reflects, in a way, the darkness I have always felt surrounds me. I love Edgar Allan Poe and his appreciation of the more macabre things in life. It is easy for one who grapples with internal dark forces to become engulfed in thinking about your own problems and wild thoughts. Reading helps me get out of my own brain and focus on something other than myself. Reading is calming and therapeutic. I have not had an extensive education up until now, so everything I know is from the books that line the shelves in my house. I'm proud of the education I have given myself, and one of the biggest goals I have in life is to take what I know and expand upon it in a university setting.

I don't spend a lot of money on clothes. I buy most of my wardrobe on Amazon, to be honest, but I do enjoy putting on a cute outfit, doing some really dramatic makeup, and feeling prideful about the way I look. My weight has fluctuated drastically over the years: I have gone from a size two to a size fourteen and back again, sometimes in a matter of months. When I am on the bigger side, I still like the curvy way I look, and when I am super skinny, this is usually a sign that I have gone through something particularly stressful. I can look hot at any size, which is something the viewers of my show don't often see. When I am filming, I am usually on the bigger side, and I don't dress that nicely. That's because I get depressed around this time for lots of reasons, mostly because it is just hard to put myself out there like I do. But when I get dressed up to go out, I can look really fly, and I think every girl, no matter how much money she has or how many pounds she weighs, should be able to feel that way too.

A while back, I decided I needed to create something that might last beyond my TV show. I decided I wanted to open an online boutique. A fan reached out to me and offered to help. I would spend hours a night looking through clothes and then I would buy them and have them sent to her house to ship out. Our online boutique was called Forever Haute. To this day, this is one of my most proud moments. For this online store, I would curate pieces of clothing that I thought would look cute on any size girl for affordable prices. I picked out really high-end pieces, nothing rated below four stars in quality from the manufacturer, and the fan and her daughter would put cute little tags on them and ship them from their house.

When the site went live, it crashed. It had so many visitors, and almost everything on the website sold out within hours. I even wore one of the dresses I had for sale on the site on the red carpet at the VMAs. There were barricades between me and the fans that night, but I busted through the partitions in my flowing blue dress to sign autographs, and I was so happy that my fans could go and buy this dress for a good price and wear it to their prom. This was a happy moment for me, and one I am going to revisit soon.

Even today, if a publication wants to talk about me, they often use the picture of me in that blue dress on the red carpet of the VMAs. Whenever I see the dress, it's a reminder that I can do anything I set my mind to. I spent over $50,000 on that clothing line, making sure all of the clothes on my website were cute and great quality. Eventually, though, with everything I would end up going through, it was too much for me to handle and I had to close down the site. I keep meaning to go back to this business because I was good at it, and I want to make my own clothes someday. It is on my list of goals, and usually, when I set a goal for myself, I achieve it.

Fat shaming on the internet is something I have to deal with often, and even though I am somewhat comfortable with my figure no matter what size I am, I can't say the harsh words from people who don't like my body doesn't hurt me. If I am looking really heavy, it is usually because I am in a depressive episode. So being called names for how I look probably feels something like a person in a wheelchair being made fun of because they can't walk. People can be mean, and heavier girls know that better than anyone. Luckily, I care more about the thoughts in people's heads than how they look, and as long as I am behaving properly and treating people with respect, I don't think it should matter how big I am. Starting a clothing line of cute clothes that fit a whole range of sizes is my way of trying to help bigger girls feel pretty, and I am excited about pursuing this career again.

The single thing that comes from my haters that hurts me the most, however, is when people criticize me as a mother. I am an easy target for those that gain pleasure from striking at public figures shaded by the anonymity of the internet, and attacking my parenting seems to be a popular way for people to attack me. Yes, I do not have full physical custody of my two children, but I share joint legal custody of both of my children with their fathers. As usual, I am not even a fraction of what I appear on camera. Nobody is simply a summation of actions. I love my children with everything I have, and they are the only reason I am still on this planet. Everything I am doing, from being sober to avoiding physical conflict, is for my children. So maybe on TV it seems like I am making bad choices or alienating my daughter, but in reality, even though I make tons of mistakes, she is always on the forefront of my brain.

I know lots of moms say the same thing. We all love our kids. And I know how we interact with them, physical custody or not, is important. We all want our kids to be happy and okay. But the difference between me and some moms is that I am pulling my pure love from the center of the typhoon that is my broken brain. So when my dedication to being a better mom to my kids is attacked, to not react in an aggressive manner requires a great deal of restraint. To be called a bad mom after all that I have struggled to overcome feels like someone stuck a knife through my chest. I never cry. I never get scared. Except when it comes to my kids.

To be a mother means to think about the well-being of your children constantly, even if it is to your own detriment. And in that way, I am no different than any mom I know. Right now, I have parenting time with my son that is typical for a noncustodial parent of any toddler. I see him on Wednesdays and every other weekend. He doesn't spend the night yet, but I hope to have him spend nights someday because I can't wait to wake up with my little Bubby and feed him breakfast in the morning. The days I have my son are the best days; I can set everything else aside and just concentrate on him. My brain magically becomes uncluttered and my other responsibilities fade to the background. Those are my favorite days.

Things with my daughter right now are not going as well. My son is only three, so he doesn't know about all of the things that surround having me as a mom. My daughter, on the other hand, has famously witnessed the ups and downs that come with being the offspring of someone who has mental health issues and who used to be addicted to drugs. It's hard to talk to children about mental illness or addiction. They just don't have the ability to understand the complexity of the reason Mommy can't get out of bed today. And I understand that, and I am really conscious of not burdening my daughter with information she is not mature enough to handle. But not making excuses for myself to her has probably hurt her opinion of me, and I have to live with that.

Also, I am aware that my daughter is at an impressionable age, and even if it is not consciously done, she is being made to choose between my ex and his wife and me. Nobody is making her choose, but there are two sides. I know she feels it. Especially when we are all not getting along. So, when she is made to choose, of course she is going to pick the people who feed her and clothe her and take care of her day in and day out. When I back out of the situation so she doesn't have to feel conflicted, I look like I am a bad mom who doesn't care enough about her daughter to see her. I can't win in this situation, but I am committed to trying to make my relationship with my ex and his wife better so my daughter doesn't feel like she has to make that choice.

A worry I have about my daughter is that mental illness has a big hereditary component. My daughter has had something like eight anxiety attacks in her eleven years of life. I am scared that she is experiencing the exact same thing I went through at her age. The only thing that gives me peace of mind is that I know she does not have to live in a house with screaming parents and an alcoholic father like I did. But I do worry about her mental stability because she reminds me so much of myself. She lives full-time with my ex and his wife. And I am sure they take good care of her. She definitely does not have to worry about where her clothes will come from or if there will be dinner on the table at night. But anxiety does not have to have a source; it can just be the luck of the brain chemical draw. So I am always thinking about her wellness in this regard.

While I feel nothing but closeness and love toward my daughter, she is going through a stage right now where she is not sure of how comfortable she is around me, and I have to respect that. She is twelve years old. She knows what she likes and dislikes, and it is not up to me to force her into anything she doesn't want to do. This can come across, however, as looking like I just don't care because I am not bothering her constantly to see me or spend time with me. It's actually the opposite. It takes a lot of restraint not to bang down my ex's door and demand the time with my daughter that I am legally due. But I don't want to see her upset or put her in a situation that makes her uncomfortable. That is just not the mom that I am.

It is heartbreaking to feel disconnected from my firstborn child. My daughter is strong-willed and whip-smart, and I love talking with her about everything under the sun. But that strength can also mean she is resolute in her mindset and I know better than to try and convince her any way other than the way she feels right now. Lately, I get the feeling those around her are not painting the best picture of me. I sense she is being turned ever so slightly against me, maybe not deliberately, but kids are smart. They pick up on the opinions and feelings of adults. And my daughter is smarter and more intuitive than most. So I feel a little helpless in this situation. I am familiar with that helpless feeling, I have encountered it my whole life, and I fight every day to have a more positive outlook about what is going on with my daughter and me.

I feel badly for my daughter because I know she is being pulled in too many directions for a girl her age. She has to read horrific things about her mother in the press, she has to deal with the notoriety that comes with being on a television show at school, and she is experiencing the hormonal shifts that come with rounding the curve toward becoming teenager. I have been noticing more and more interference in her life, and I feel powerless to change that. Being on TV is my job for now, and it is how I pay my bills and support my two children. I am happy for all the time we spent together before I went to jail and after, and I know we will have closeness again. But our situation, like everything else in my life, is complicated and a work in progress.

That's why I am happy I have the time that I have with my son, who is too young to be affected by the publicity that surrounds me. We have the loveliest days together when I can see him. He loves when I give him happy cupcakes, which are really just muffins, and I love to watch him shake his little bum around and drop it low to the ground just like his Mommy. He wants to take karate because he sees me working so hard at it, and I have no doubt this little guy will surpass me in belts before I know it.

I have to drive an hour from my house to pick up my son and drop him off, and that just seems like wasted time when we could be hanging out together watching our favorite videos in our pajamas. I'm also scared of driving in bad weather, which makes it appear I don't want to see my son. The media latches on to this persona too. The headlines read: "Amber Portwood

Cancels on Seeing her Son Because of Rain!" and I know there is nothing good that can come of that. I have confidence, however, that I will prevail in our custody mediation and eventually get more time, maybe even overnights, with the little man. And those will be the best days of them all.

Spending time with my children has always done wonders for my mental state. When I am with them, my mind is clear and sharp. I find it easy to focus on them, and I have never really had any psychiatric issues when I am with them, even before I found the balance and care that makes me able to stand tall and function normally today. One of the reasons I love being with both of them is because they seem to make my own problems melt away. With my children, I am strong and clear-minded, and this has always brought me so much joy, even when things were difficult for me.

The days I spend with my son remind me of days I used to spend with my daughter before things got bad for me. I loved going to the theater when I was a little girl. I went on a school trip to see *The Nutcracker* and I thought it was the most beautiful thing I had ever seen. I shushed all the other kids so I could hear what was going on during the performance. My daughter was the same way. She loved going to shows and plays, and I loved taking her. One time I took her to the dinosaur exhibit at the Natural History Museum. She was a shy and reserved kid, so when she opened up and rode on the T. rex that moved, it was so funny to watch. When we went to the museum, she was nine years old. I told her she could have anything she wanted from the gift shop and I was so proud of her when she picked a book, not a toy.

I also took her to the fair in Indiana, and she asked me if she could have her face painted. She wanted to look like a cat. The line was so long. We waited forty-five minutes, and I remember being so proud of her that she just stood in that line waiting patiently, reading her book, while all the other kids around us complained to their parents about having to wait. Even I was annoyed at the long wait. I looked at her with her nose in a book and thought to myself, *I have a really special kid. I am so lucky.* Moments of peace and gratitude like that in my life are so fleeting that I never forget them.

When it comes to my daughter today, however, now I am the one who has to wait. I wait for her to come around. I wait for her to grow older and understand I never meant her any harm or confusion. I wait for her to realize there are two sides to every story and that the only two hearts that matter in this are hers and mine. I know my love for her shines through all that has happened and what has been told to her. I am confident enough in what we have between us, our secret and unbreakable bond, to know that someday she will come back to me. It is shattering and unspeakably hard, but—improving myself every day so that when she does come back she is prouder of me than ever—I wait.

CHAPTER

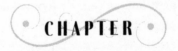

People say, take off the makeup.
You're still ugly or beautiful without it.
I believe you can be ugly or beautiful with it.
Looking at that ceiling fan, or watermill.
It is whatever I want it to be.

I'M NOT LIVING IN MY own house, the house I saved up for four years to buy with cash, because my ex is living there with my son. Unlike public perception of me, I have always cared more about my kids' happiness than my own. It's heartbreaking, though, not to live there right now because my grandma helped me pick that house out and because that kind of money, for that kind of house, in that kind of neighborhood is an accomplishment, especially coming from the life I lived when I was a little girl. So I rent a little place to lay my head, and I dream of the day when I can live in my own home, have visits with both of my children, and feel safe and complete at last.

A few years ago, right smack-dab in the middle of my quest for knowledge, enlightenment, sobriety, and universal truths, I met a cute Belgian boy online. I say boy, but he is a man. A real man who, surprisingly enough, treats me with kindness despite my many, many suitcases of baggage. He is a mailman in Belgium, and he wears a cute little uniform and makes enough money to support himself, but not much more than that. He speaks with a strong accent and needs to use Google Translate to have a conversation with me, but I think he is the funniest person ever. He came to see me in Indiana and we hit it off in person even better than we did during our long-distance banter. We spent some time together, and then COVID-19 hit. He is back in Belgium, so we have been communicating exclusively over the phone and computer for more than a year. Thanks to COVID, but also to my newfound self-imposed relationship guidelines, we are taking it slow.

I get a lot of flak about my choice in partners, especially from my mom and my brother. The problem is, I just cannot stand dating normal people. I can't imagine dating "Bob from Cleveland who works at the Stop & Shop and has been with exactly two women and is going to night school for bike maintenance." I am sure Bob is a perfectly lovely man, and I know he will make some lucky girl a great husband, but I am a powerful and dynamic person, and I need my partner to be interesting and different.

Whenever I think about my choice in partners, a song from Tech N9ne comes to mind. It's called "I Caught Crazy! (4Ever)" and the general message is that nobody is actually okay; we've all got a screw or two loose.

The bottom line is, I agree with Tech9. If you say you don't have a little crazy in you, are you really being authentic? What I like most about my Belgian friend is that he is not trying to be anything he isn't. He is weird and unusual, and those are my types of people. My Belgian mailman is interesting maybe just because he speaks beautiful French, and he never really understands what I am talking about.

I like to call my Belgian lover Pretty Dick, for obvious reasons. He calls me Baby Love. I think I introduced him to a whole new world, sexually speaking, because when I first met him, he didn't really love to give oral sex. But after a while, he couldn't get enough of giving it to me. I also grabbed his neck once during sex and he apparently liked that. So, overall, I think it is safe to say I opened a few doors for him that he probably didn't even know existed. When he came to visit me from Belgium for Thanksgiving, he met my family and I know they had no idea what to do with him. Which, of course, just made me like him more.

We haven't put a label on our relationship. It ebbs and flows like most relationships do, but minus the heated exchanges of my past relationships—just in a smooth up-and-down fashion that feels comfortable and nurturing to me. I don't feel the need to be in a serious relationship right now, but I think everyone likes to have someone to talk to, and in this regard, I am just like everyone else. Also, I am in love with him, and there is really no talking me out of that.

I feel confident this man does not want anything from me other than love, which is a refreshing change from my three serious boyfriends, all of whom broke my heart and my trust in one form or another. The mailman passed a lie detector test, so right there I have traded up from my ex-fiancé, at least. He has already saved up $7,000 to come here and spend time with me when the pandemic is over, which I think is sweet. Also, if he is after me for fame or money, he sure is playing the long game. I haven't seen him in person in over a year, and I certainly have learned my lesson about sharing bank accounts and money with anyone, maybe ever again. So I don't think there is any question of whether he is with me for that or not.

People like to tell me on social media that they know my Belgian mailman friend has been messaging girls or that girls send him naked pictures of themselves, and I just laugh. I get sent a lot of pictures, too, from men and women. We have sat together and gone over all the pictures we have been sent, laughing and turned on at the same time. I know getting hit on over the internet comes with the territory for two people in the public eye like we are, so it doesn't bother me. As for talking to girls, he says he doesn't, but I guess it doesn't really matter either. We are not in a relationship: we can both do what we want to do. I have been cheated on so much in my life I am almost numb to it at this point, and I certainly do not put myself in a position to be hurt as easily as I used to. It took a while, but I am growing up.

One of the characteristics of a borderline personality is a very active libido, and I have that in spades. When I used to experience manic phases of bipolar, sex was a big part of my mania. Because my medication is so carefully monitored now, I am able to curb my desires—well, that and the fact that the medications kill my sex drive to a degree. I am learning to try and do everything in moderation, and sex is no exception.

This year, because of COVID-19, I have become almost a full-on recluse, and it has been nice to slow down and notice the things in life that release just as many endorphins as sex and drugs. I have been forced, because of COVID and the oceans that separate us, to be away from my Belgian sweetheart for a year now, and it has done nothing but strengthen our romantic friendship. It has been enlightening to watch a relationship with a man unfold in such a nonsexual manner. I never knew I had the capacity to relate this well to a lover without having sex with him constantly.

My love of music is well documented because it is hard for me not to talk about the songs and musicians that rock my world—literally. I love all kinds of music, from classical to hard rock, hip-hop to rap, and nothing turns me on more than hearing just the right song at just the right time. I love to sing; all the girls on *Teen Mom* would make me sing for them during breaks in filming. I think having things we enjoy and that we are good at is so important for those afflicted with any kind of mental illness. We are all searching for ways out of our madness, and for me, music is that way out.

It is a strange time to be alive nowadays, with the world stopped. It's odd not seeing the man I am dating for a year due to COVID, and I find myself canceling on seeing my son more often than I would like because I am scared of getting him sick. There are no parties to go to. I am not frequenting restaurants or seeing friends. But I have to say the quiet of the past year has helped me center myself and focus on taking the medicine that keeps me sane and the things I must do every day to help me advance to the next.

Being bipolar and also having borderline personality disorder comes with many behaviors that are hard to catch and correct when I am by myself all the time. In the past, a boyfriend would notice I was going into a manic phase, or my mom would point out that I hadn't left my bed for three days. Nowadays it is just me looking for the signs of the next major mood adjustment and trying to keep my head above water when I am positive I am going to drown. I am strong, independent, and well educated on my host of mental issues, but it is usually difficult to see that you are in a tailspin until the damage to yourself or someone else is already done. Thankfully, I have finally learned to lean on professionals and medication designed to help people like me, and I have learned techniques to stop my illnesses in their tracks, so I don't really need anyone else looking out for me.

One program that has really helped me has been the batterers intervention program. Maybe it was the timing of it all. I was finally ready to accept responsibility for my actions and learn ways to keep the actions from happening again. Whatever the reason, I learned a lot from this program. They teach you the power of holding back and the value of walking away from conflict. Where I grew up, it was a sign of weakness to walk away from a fight. This program taught me that walking away from a potentially explosive situation is actually a sign of great inner strength.

Because I am a high-profile case, I got lucky enough to warrant the head of the Indiana Batterers Intervention Program as my personal coach. I have meetings with him every week, sometimes twice a week, and it feels like bonus therapy. During these meetings, we talk a lot about my past and where all this pent-up anger comes from. I have learned that it is okay to feel angry. Of course some girl yelling at me that I am a trash human and should kill myself is going to make me mad. But it is what you do with that anger that matters, and for over two years now, I have been learning ways to channel my anger that do not involve striking other people. This has seriously been life changing for me.

Recently, I applied and was accepted to attend online classes at Purdue University Global. I had first attempted to apply to Indiana University, imagining myself attending classes during the day while my son was in school, in some other life. But they asked about my criminal record and I lost interest in going to a college that cares about that sort of thing. I am going to get my

Bachelor of Science in psychology and behavioral analysis, and I could not be more excited. This is a goal of mine that seems more attainable than ever, with my clear (ish) mind and some time on my hands, so I am planning on applying myself to this degree with everything I have left over from fighting my mental illnesses.

My parents did not have college degrees, so it will be a big deal in my family when I complete this degree and go on to study neurology. My brother went to college and is now a corrections officer at a prison in Florida, which is funny since his sister was in jail. But I am so proud of him for emerging from the battlefield that was our childhood and making something of himself, and I want to follow in his footsteps.

My psychiatrist calls me a true empath, and when he first told me that, so many things in my life made sense. Being an empath kind of means you take on all the feelings of the people around you. Through listening to a person or seeing how they act, I can feel another person's feelings so deeply it is as if I am that person myself. Being an empath is not easy. I take on so much of the pain around me that it can hurt me physically and inflict wounds on my psyche, and much of what I talk to my psychiatrist about centers around lessening the pain I feel for others.

My mom has been seeing a psychiatrist for a year now too. She was having trouble processing her own mom's death last year. My mom told me that a while back she had mentioned to her back doctor's wife that she was having some trouble processing troubling memories that she had, so she sent her to the psychiatrist that she is seeing now. It broke my heart to hear this because I love my mom more than anyone in the world. I hate to think of her struggling or in pain in any way. But I am obviously a firm believer in therapy, and I am glad to hear she is talking to someone on a regular basis that can help her. It can't be easy to be my mom.

I always feel like in fighting my mental illnesses, I am playing a game of football that never ends. I am the quarterback, and I run and get tackled and I throw the ball, but all I want to do is sit down on the sidelines and take a rest. That break never comes, however. You are always playing, constantly battling, and you never, ever get to rest. This is why it was always funny to me when people would call me lazy. Yes, I used to lie down a lot. My medications all made me tired, and it was exhausting battling demons all day long. I used to experience such severe bouts of depression that I would have to lie down to stop myself from running off of a bridge. My nights were filled with psychosis and visions that didn't allow me to get much sleep, so I might have been just tired from being up three nights in a row. Even now that I am doing all the things, I need to so that I am well. I can still say one thing for sure: there is nothing lazy about living with these conditions.

Before I cleared my mind and dedicated myself to my regiment of therapy, medication, and calming methods, I would think about killing myself pretty much on a daily basis. I would get upset about not being with my kids every day and think *what is the point of living?* There is nothing more dangerous than a mentally ill person with nothing to lose. Even without any of those dark thoughts, I still always get anxious when I am about to film my show. I am always worried about the public's perception of me after my show has aired, and it gives me crippling anxiety.

I am on a pretty strict regimen for my probation this time around. I must attend classes, submit drug tests, fill out paperwork, and submit writing assignments on a regular basis. I have a year left of this, and then my felony conviction is changed to a misdemeanor and I can go on with my life. This sounds like a surmountable obstacle, but in reality, the idea of being unwatched and unchecked is concerning. A few years ago, I got a new car, and I knew I needed tags and plates for it, so I just took them off my old car and put them on the new one. I drove around like that for a year until my brother noticed. When he told me every new car needs a new set of tags, I was shocked. This is just an example of how being on a television show since I was seventeen years old has sheltered me from the responsibilities of being a true adult. I have no idea what will happen to me financially when the show ends for me. I know, however, that I will take everything I have learned in the past few years about my mental health and apply it to living a good life.

In the end, I feel I was put on this earth to help people who have suffered in the same way that I am. I would like to become a neurologist so I can study the brain and find ways to help treat mental illness. I would love to open a halfway house to help someone who is an addict transition back into society from rehab or jail. I would like to give talks and seminars to talk about what I have learned about mental illness, especially to young people so they can get the help they need before they make the mistakes that I made in my life. I want people to know that mental illness is something we cannot change. It is as much a part of us as the color of our eyes. But there are things everyone can do to control these illnesses and live a happy, healthy, and normal life. It is important for me to share that with the world.

In this book, I have only told a fraction of my real story. I have too much integrity to tear down other people by telling truths that put myself in a better light at the expense of others. There is so much more to every story that would make my behavior make more sense and that I wish people knew. But it was important to me to shed light on mental illness because I truly believe these disorders should be talked about in the light of day and in detail more often. So I wrote what I can talk about that is personal to me, and that is it. I hope it is enough to bring about change, I really do. That is all that matters.

I believe in past lives, and I think you can live a few different lives within the one you are living now. I feel like I have lived many lives already, and I am only thirty-one years old. I look at the troubles of the past decade or so as one past life of mine, and I know all of the good things to come will be my new life. Stronger relationships with my children, a career in medicine, reading and writing more—all of these things will fill my days the way fighting and drugs filled my days when I am younger.

I have a lot to do, I tell myself, and I have people who depend on me. And so I soldier on, darting and dodging life's curveballs, living in my little box, waiting for the glimpse of sunlight, such as a day spent dancing and singing with my son or a night spent on the phone with my daughter, to help me out of the darkness. I am a strong person, I will persevere, and I will accomplish things nobody expects of me. I might not be completely normal, but I am going to do great things.

I am excited to become a therapist, psychiatrist, or even a neurologist. The possibilities are limitless with the right education and the drive to make a real change in the world. With my studies at the university, I am starting to gather the tools I need to begin the next phase of my life. I have been through so much, but I am confident I can use what I have learned to help other people. I know it is what I was put on the earth to do, and I am just getting started. Every second of this crazy life has led to this moment: closing the chapters that came before and beginning a new one. This is the end of the story of my life so far, but I know in my heart it is just the beginning of the life I was meant to live.

MENTAL HEALTH RESOURCES

1. National Alliance on Mental Illness (NAMI): https://www.nami.org
2. National Institute of Mental Health (NIH): https://www.nimh.nih.gov
3. The JED Foundation: https://www.jedfoundation.org
4. Depression and Bipolar Support Alliance (DBSA): https://www.dbsalliance.org
5. Mental Health Is Health: https://mentalhealthishealth.us
6. Teen Health and Wellness: https://teenhealthandwellness.com
7. Substance Abuse and Mental Health Services Administration (SAMHSA): https://www.samhsa.gov
8. Dual Recovery Anonymous: http://www.draonline.org
9. The Bipolar Child: https://bipolarchild.com

RECOMMENDED READING

1. *Manic* by Terri Cheney
2. *An Unquiet Mind* by Kay Redfield Jamison
3. *The Bipolar Child: The Definitive and Reassuring Guide to Childhood's Most Misunderstood Disorder* by Demitri F. Papolos, M.D., and Janice Papolos
4. *Loving Someone with Bipolar Disorder* by Julie A. Fast and John D. Preston, PsyD
5. *Surviving Manic Depression: A Manual on Bipolar Disorder for Patients, Families and Providers* by E. Fuller Torrey, M.D., and Michael B. Knable, D.O.
6. *Stop Walking on Eggshells: Taking Your Life Back When Someone You Care About Has Borderline Personality Disorder* by Paul T. Mason, M.S., and Randi Kreger
7. *Bipolar Disorder for Dummies* by Candida Fink, M.D., and Joe Kraynak, M.A.
8. *The Enchiridion* by Epictetus
9. *The Frenzy of Renown* by Leo Braudy

ABOUT THE AUTHOR

A MBER PORTWOOD WAS CAST IN the reality television series *16 and Pregnant* in 2009, and has since catapulted to infamy for her several run-ins with the law that included a 17-month stint in prison. She is the mother of two children, and currently stars on the show *Teen Mom OG,* where her controversial life plays out weekly to a devoted audience. She is the author of NEVER TOO LATE, is currently attending Purdue University Global, and is an outspoken advocate for mental health and wellness.

ACKNOWLEDGMENTS

I DEDICATE THIS BOOK TO ALL of the family, friends, and supporters in my life. I also want the naysayers to take a glimpse at the lives of people with mental illnesses. This book isn't really here to change your minds because the majority of you are always going to be assholes, but now you're much more educated assholes, at least in this subject. Thank you to everyone in my life—too many to say, honestly—that pushed me to be better and rethink my ways. Your wisdom and support will always be with me.

Sending all my love,
Amber

*And a special thank you to Elissa and Thea for being the badass women they are. Nothing would have been possible without you. Love you, bitches.